Let's Talk About Sex

CHANGING BODIES, GROWING UP, SEX and SEXUAL HEALTH

PRAISE FOR
Let's Talk About Sex

"A great book… All the facts are there without reservation, but it has a gentle approach that is very reassuring."
The Times Educational Supplement

"An everything-you-always-wanted-to-know guide that is clear and cheerful."
The Independent on Sunday

"Informative, down-to-earth and humorous, containing everything a pre-teen will want to know about growing up – the best book I have seen on this subject."
Nanette Newman in **The Sunday Express**

"I was impressed by the brave and comprehensive coverage of the subject."
Judith Hann in **The Guardian**

"A wonderful new book for 10- to 14-year-olds."
She

"It's perfect for pre-teenage kids and teenagers. And you may even discover a few facts of life you never knew!"
Best

"An excellent guide for 10- to 14-year-olds. It covers sensitive topics like conception, babies, puberty, family and birth control in a frank and lively way."
Essentials

"An excellent read … it makes learning fun and is very easy to understand."
Shout Magazine

"A child will no doubt find this book very readable … the style is matter-of-fact, informative and responsible. It does not preach or talk down to the young reader."
The School Librarian

"*Let's Talk About Sex* is very much the star of the show. The cartoons are non-threatening… This unselfconscious approach, rippling with gentle humour, eases readers into what could have been potentially embarrassing situations."
Books for Keeps

"A straightforward guide to puberty for 10- to 14-year olds, covering facts and feelings in almost equal measure. The text is serious, with an agreeable tone that is factual without being pedantic. The illustrations capture a similar balance by being humorous but not trivial."
The Bookseller

"Its straightforward, unembarrassed, and unpatronizing approach is exactly what children and young adults need in their quest for accurate information – but cartoons and line drawings make it friendly rather than dauntingly clinical."
Time Out

"Outstanding."
Junior Education

★ "A wonderful guide for young adolescents setting sail on the stormy seas of puberty."
School Library Journal (*starred review*)

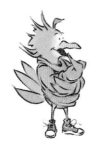

A Note to the Reader

Celebrating the Twentieth Anniversary Edition
of Let's Talk About Sex

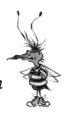

Ever since *Let's Talk About Sex* was first published twenty years ago, we have never stopped talking with children, teens, and adults about the information and issues in this book. This has given us the opportunity and privilege to learn even more about what you – children and teens – need to know to stay healthy.

Over the years, we have also continued to ask experts, including parents, teachers, librarians, doctors, nurses, psychologists, psychoanalysts, scientists and clergy, what information about puberty, sex and sexual health needs to be changed, updated or added to keep you healthy. Whenever changes in the text and the art are necessary to make this book as up-to-date and accurate as possible, we make them.

For this twentieth anniversary edition, we have updated the scientific and medical information about reproduction, birth control, abortion, sexual abuse and sexually transmitted diseases, including HIV/AIDS. And we have included information about gender identity.

Since so many of you use mobile phones, tablets and computers to go online to find information and to communicate with others, we have also added more information about the benefits and risks of being online. We believe this will help you use the Internet to find accurate and responsible information about sexual health and will also help you protect your own as well as your friends' and your family's personal safety.

While writing and illustrating this book, we checked and rechecked the scientific information and the latest research. What we learned from scientists and health professionals is that knowledge about this subject is continually evolving and changing. While there is much agreement, there is also some disagreement, and some questions still remain. At this time, the information in this book is as up-to-date and as accurate as possible. But if you have more questions or need further information, most always it can be very helpful to talk with someone you know and trust – a parent, doctor, nurse, teacher, school counsellor, therapist or clergy member.

Today, even more children have a chance to read *Let's Talk About Sex*, as it has been translated into more than thirty-five languages and continues to be used around the world – from the United States to the United Kingdom to Denmark to the Netherlands, from Germany to Italy to Spain to Poland, from Japan to Taiwan to Mongolia to South Africa.

We hope that our newest edition will help to keep you – our next generation of children and teens – healthy and safe. We also hope it will help you and your friends make informed and responsible decisions about sexual health as you continue to grow up and go through puberty and adolescence.

Robie H. Harris and Michael Emberley

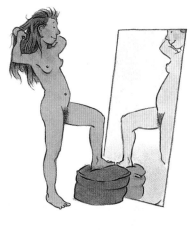

Let's Talk About Sex

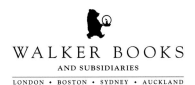

A Book About Changing Bodies,
Growing Up, Sex and Sexual Health

Written by
ROBIE H. HARRIS
Illustrated by
MICHAEL EMBERLEY

WALKER BOOKS
AND SUBSIDIARIES
LONDON · BOSTON · SYDNEY · AUCKLAND

Contents

INTRODUCTION
Lots of Questions

Changing Bodies, Growing Up, Sex and Sexual Health   1

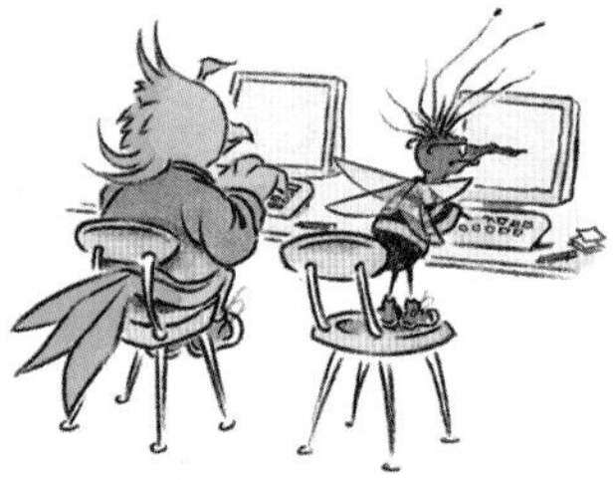

PART ONE
What Is Sex?

1 Girl or Boy, Female or Male   2
Sex and Gender

2 Making Babies   3
Sexual Reproduction

3 Strong Feelings   4
Sexual Desire

4 Making Love   6
Sexual Intercourse

5 Who You Are   8
Straight, Lesbian, Gay,
Bisexual, Transgender

PART TWO
Our Bodies

6 The Human Body   12
All Kinds of Bodies

7 Outside and Inside   16
The Female Sex Organs

8 Outside and Inside   19
The Male Sex Organs

9 Words   22
Talking about Bodies and Sex

PART THREE
Puberty

10 Changes and Messages   24
Puberty and Hormones

11 The Travels of the Egg   27
Female Puberty

12 The Travels of the Sperm   32
Male Puberty

13 Not All at Once!   36
Growing and Changing Bodies

14 More Changes!   38
Taking Care of Your Body

15 Back and Forth,   40
Up and Down
New and Changing Feelings

16 Perfectly Normal   43
Masturbation

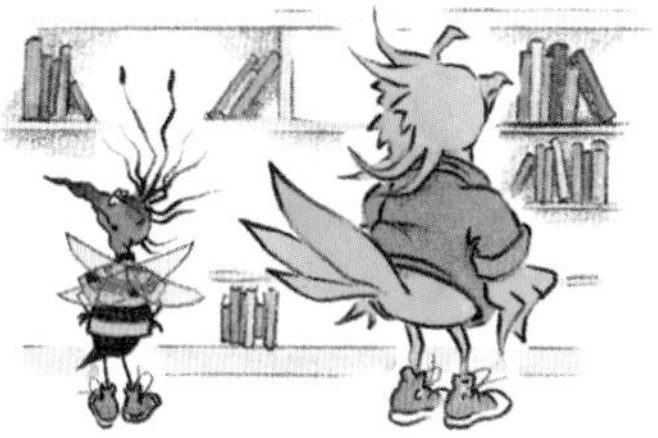

PART FOUR
Families and Babies

17 All Sorts of Families   45
Taking Care of Babies and Children

18 Instructions from   48
Mum and Dad
The Cell: Genes and Chromosomes

19 A Kind of Sharing   50
Cuddling, Kissing, Touching,
and Sexual Intercourse

20 Before Birth   54
Pregnancy

21 What a Trip!   58
Birth

22 Other Arrivals   62
More Ways to Have a
Baby and Family

PART FIVE
Decisions

23 Planning Ahead   65
Postponement, Abstinence
and Contraception

24 Laws and Rulings   71
Abortion

PART SIX
Staying Healthy

25 Helpful – Fun – Creepy –   74
Dangerous
Texting, Messaging, Emailing,
Being Online

26 Talk About It   80
Sexual Abuse

27 Getting a Check-up   83
Sexually Transmitted Diseases

28 Scientists Working   86
Day and Night
HIV and AIDS

29 Staying Healthy   90
Responsible Choices

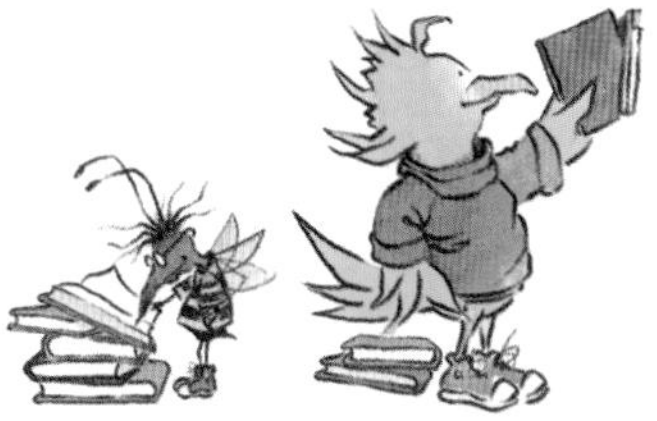

The Bird and the Bee

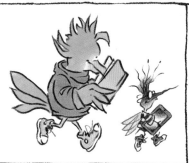

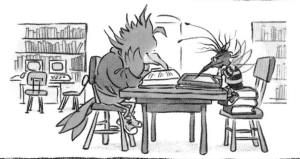

Hey! Do you want to know what I'm reading?

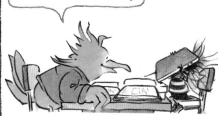

No. Not now. I'm in the middle of a book about astronomy.

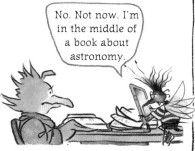

I'm reading a science book too, you know.

You are! Well, that's a first!

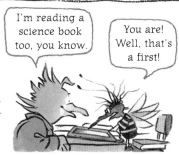

This book will be a first for you. Take a look. I guarantee you will like it.

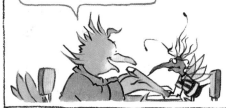

Oh ... my goodness! This is a book on...

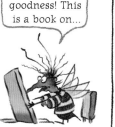

Sex. You have a problem with that?

I certainly do! I'll stick to the stars, thank you.

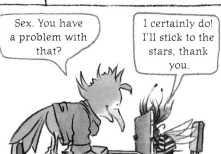

You're a chicken.

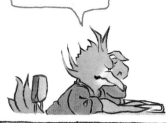

Have you lost your mind? I'm a bee. And bees are extremely brave.

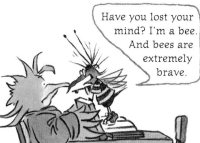

If that's true, then take a look at this book.

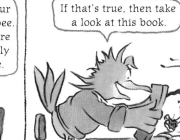

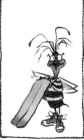

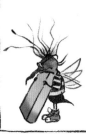

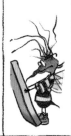

Well, OK, but just a quick look.

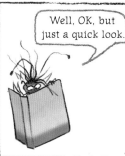

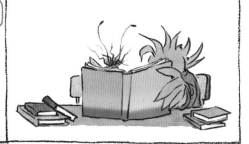

INTRODUCTION
Lots of Questions

Changing Bodies, Growing Up, Sex and Sexual Health

Some time between the ages of eight or nine and fifteen or so, children's bodies begin to change and grow into adult bodies.

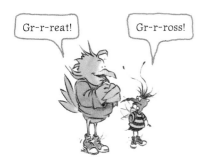

Most young people wonder about and have lots of questions about what will be happening to them as their bodies change and grow during this time.

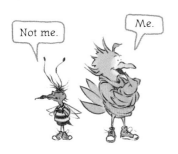

It's perfectly normal for people to be curious about and want to know about their changing and growing bodies. Most of the changes – but not all – that take place during this time make it possible for humans to make and give birth to a baby. And making a baby has a lot to do with sex.

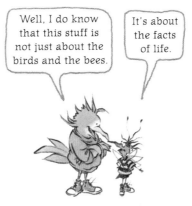

Sex is about a lot of things – bodies, growing up, families, babies, love, caring, curiosity, feelings, respect, responsibility, biology and health. There are times when sickness and danger can be a part of sex, too.

Most young people wonder about and have lots of questions about sex. It's also perfectly normal to want to know about sex.

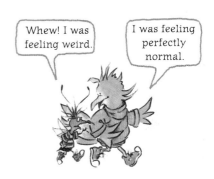

You may wonder why it's a good idea to learn some facts about bodies, about growing up, about sex and about sexual health. It's important because these facts can help you stay healthy, take good care of yourself and make good decisions about yourself as you are growing up and for the rest of your life.

Besides, learning about these things can be fascinating and fun.

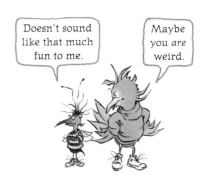

PART ONE

What Is Sex?

1

Girl or Boy, Female or Male
Sex and Gender

What is sex? What is it ... exactly? What is it all about?

These are questions lots of young people wonder about. You needn't feel embarrassed or stupid if you don't know the answers, because sex is not a simple matter.

Sex is many things, and people have many different feelings and opinions about it. That's why there is more than one answer to the question, what is sex?

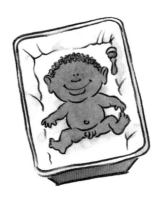

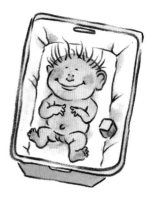

One way to find out about sex is to ask someone you know and trust. Remember, there are no stupid questions. Another way to find out about sex is to read about it. For example, you can look up the meaning of the word *sex* in the dictionary.

Here is what one dictionary says under the word *sex*:

> **1**: *Either of the two main groups, female or male, into which living things are placed.*

People always want to

know the sex of a new baby. So it's no surprise that – even if the parent or parents knew the sex of the baby before birth – the moment a baby is born, someone always seems to shout out, "It's a GIRL!" or "It's a BOY!"

And usually one of the first

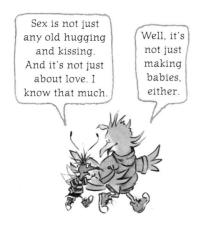

Sex is not just any old hugging and kissing. And it's not just about love. I know that much.

Well, it's not just making babies, either.

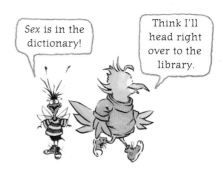

Sex is in the dictionary!

Think I'll head right over to the library.

questions children ask when they hear that a new child is joining their class is, "Is it a girl or a boy?"

When people use the word *sex* in this way, they are usually talking about what gender someone is – whether a person is female or male, a girl or a boy, a woman or a man.

Gender is another word for whether a person is male or female. Gender is also about the thoughts and feelings a person has about being a female or about being a male.

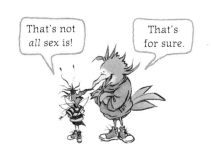

2
Making Babies
Sexual Reproduction

The dictionary tells us more about sex. It says:

2: *Sexual Reproduction.*

Sex is also about reproduction – making babies. *To reproduce* means to *produce again*, or *make again*.

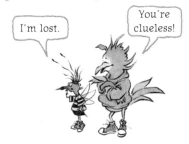

Certain parts of our bodies make it possible for a male and a female, when their bodies have grown up, to reproduce – to make babies. The parts of our bodies that make this possible are called the reproductive organs.

Our bodies' organs are the parts of our bodies that have special jobs to perform. For example, the heart is the organ whose special job is to pump blood. Scientists know that most organs inside our bodies, such as our hearts, our lungs and our stomachs, are the same whether we are male or female. One group of organs that is not the same for a female and a male is the reproductive organs.

People also call the reproductive organs the sexual organs or the sex organs. The female and male sex organs are designed to work in an amazingly interesting way. They are different from each other because they have different jobs to do.

Both males and females have outer sex organs and inner

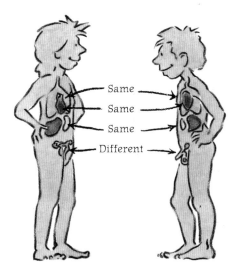

sex organs. Some are located between our legs and are on the outside of our bodies. Some are tucked inside our bodies. The sex organs on the outside of a person's body are often called the genitals, and the sex organs on the inside of a person's body are called the reproductive organs.

If you are female, your vagina and ovaries are two of your sex organs. If you are male, your penis and testicles are two of your sex organs.

When the word *sex* is used in this way, people are talking either about the female and male sex organs or about making a new human being – making a baby.

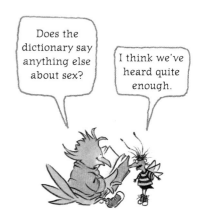

Does the dictionary say anything else about sex?

I think we've heard quite enough.

3
Strong Feelings
Sexual Desire

The dictionary tells us even more about sex. It says:

3: *Sexual Desire.*

Sex is also about the desire to be physically close to someone, as close as you can be.

Do you ever really want or crave something? That's desire, like when you really want someone to be your best friend or when you really want chocolate ice cream.

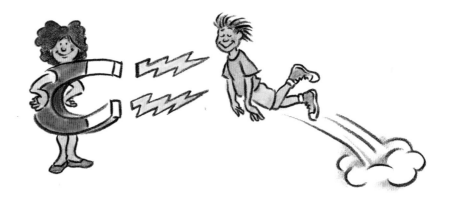

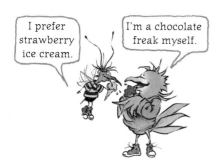

I prefer strawberry ice cream.

I'm a chocolate freak myself.

You don't know why you want these things. You don't even think about why you want them. You just want them. These are simply feelings of wanting – of desire.

Sexual desire is different from these desires – different from just wanting chocolate ice cream, or wanting someone to be your best friend, or even wanting to snuggle up to your mum or dad, a friend, a pet or a cuddly toy.

Sexual desire means you feel attracted to someone in a very strong way: like being pulled by a magnet. You want to be as physically close to that person as you can be.

Even though you may think about that person a lot, sexual desire is mostly the way you feel in your body about that person. Your body may feel excited or warm or quivery or tingly. And sometimes these feelings can be very strong.

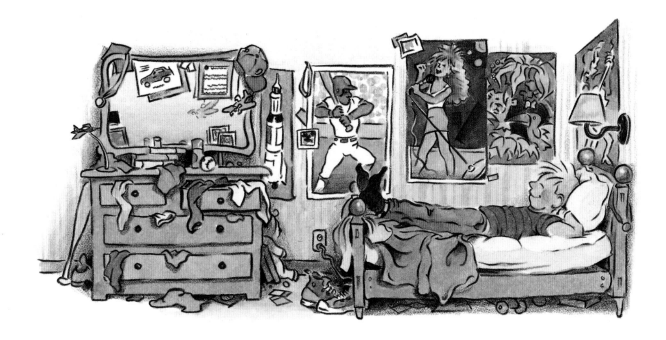

For lots of young people, part of sexual desire can be the fun of chasing and teasing or having a crush on someone. Often it's hard to stop thinking about that person, and you may even think you are in love with him or her. That's called "having a crush" on someone.

Both girls and boys have crushes. They have crushes on people they know, as well as on people they don't know – like television or film stars, pop singers or sports celebrities.

They have crushes on people of the same sex, as well as on people of the opposite sex, on people who are the same age, older, or younger. Having a crush on someone is perfectly normal.

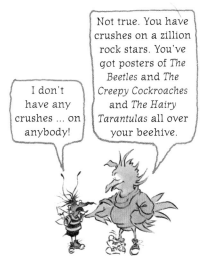

I don't have any crushes ... on anybody!

Not true. You have crushes on a zillion rock stars. You've got posters of *The Beetles* and *The Creepy Cockroaches* and *The Hairy Tarantulas* all over your beehive.

The feelings and thoughts you may have about other people and their bodies can make you feel very excited. Some people call this "feeling sexy".

Some of you are probably noticing the changes in your own bodies and the differences between your body and your friends' bodies. Sex can also be about the many new thoughts and feelings you may have about what's happening to you and your body as you are growing up.

4
Making Love
Sexual Intercourse

The dictionary tells us one more thing about sex. It says:

4: *Sexual Intercourse.*

Sex also means sexual intercourse. Some people call sexual intercourse "having sex".

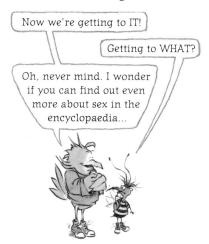

Now we're getting to IT!

Getting to WHAT?

Oh, never mind. I wonder if you can find out even more about sex in the encyclopaedia...

Sexual intercourse happens when two people – a female and a male or two females or two males – feel very sexy and very attracted to each other and want to be very close to each other in a sexual way. When a female and a male are so close that the male's penis goes inside the female's vagina, the vagina stretches open in a way that fits around the penis.

When this happens, it is possible for a female and a male – once their reproductive organs have grown up – to make a baby.

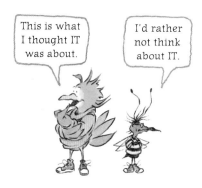

This is what I thought IT was about.

I'd rather not think about IT.

Most people don't have sexual intercourse only when they want to make a baby.

Most often, people have sexual intercourse because it feels good. People have sexual intercourse well into old age.

People also call sexual intercourse "making love" or "love-making", because it's a way of expressing love. But sexual intercourse is only one way of expressing love.

Hugging, cuddling, holding hands, kissing and touching are other ways of expressing love. So is just being with someone you like a lot and telling that person, "I love you".

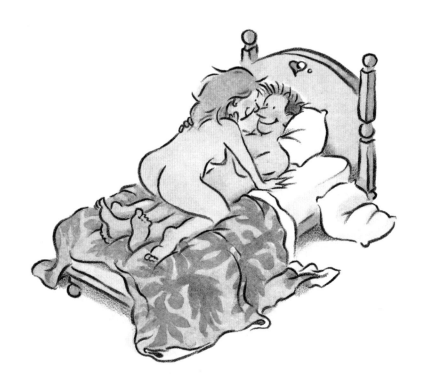

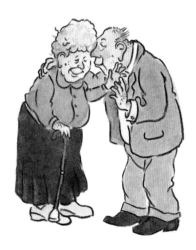
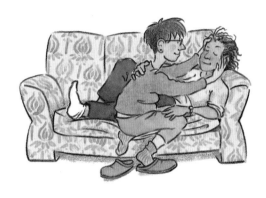
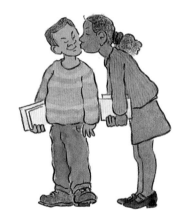

There are some things about sex and sexual intercourse that are important to know and remember:

- It makes sense to wait to have sexual intercourse until you are old enough and responsible enough to make healthy decisions about sex.
- Every female and every male has the right to say no to any kind of touching – even when one person is older, or a lot older, or stronger, or a lot stronger than the other person.
- A relationship that includes sexual contact often comes with complicated feelings.
- Sexual intercourse – "having sex" – can involve the penis and the vagina, or the mouth and the genitals, or the penis and the anus.
- After sexual intercourse that involves the vagina and the penis, the female can become pregnant. But there are ways that people can help protect themselves from having a baby.
- During sexual intercourse, serious infections – such as HIV, the virus that causes AIDS – as well as other infections that are less serious, can be passed from one person to the other. However, there are ways in which people can help protect themselves from getting or passing on these infections.

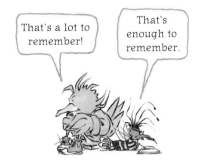

That's a lot to remember!

That's enough to remember.

So sex is a lot of things – even feelings and thoughts.

Sex is the desire to be very close to someone.

Sex is touching the sexual parts of the body.

Sex is intercourse.

Sex is making babies.

And sex is whether you are male or female.

Sometimes people use the word *sexuality* to talk about sex. When people use the word *sexuality*, they are usually talking about everything in our daily lives that makes us sexual human beings – our gender, our sexual feelings, thoughts and desires, as well as any sexual contact, from sexual touching to sexual intercourse.

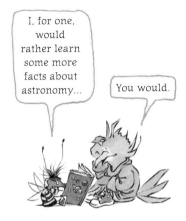

I, for one, would rather learn some more facts about astronomy...

You would.

5
Who You Are
Straight, Lesbian, Gay, Bisexual, Transgender

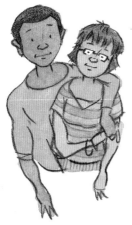 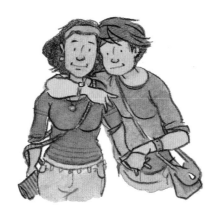 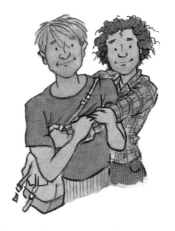

Straight, lesbian, gay and *bisexual* are words that have to do with sexual desire and sex.

A person who is straight is someone who is sexually attracted to people of the opposite sex, or, as some say, the other sex. Heterosexual is another name for a straight person. *Heteros* is the ancient Greek word for *other*.

a male and a female – are attracted to, may fall in love with, or may have a sexual relationship with each other.

A person who is gay is someone who is sexually attracted to people of the same sex. Homosexual is another name for a gay person. *Homos* is the ancient Greek word for *same*. In a gay relationship, two people of the same sex – a male

and a male, or a female and a female – are attracted to, may fall in love with, and may have a sexual relationship with each other.

A gay relationship between two females is also called a lesbian relationship. The word *lesbian* began to be used in the late nineteenth century. It refers to the time, about 600 B.C., when the great female poet Sappho

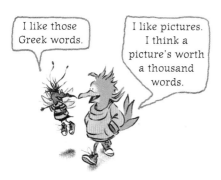

I like those Greek words.

I like pictures. I think a picture's worth a thousand words.

In a straight relationship, two people of opposite sexes –

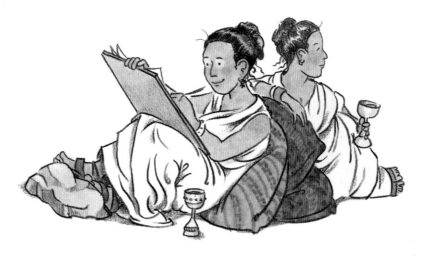

lived on the Greek island of Lesbos. Sappho wrote about friendship and love between women.

The ancient Greeks thought that love between two men was the highest form of love. In the ancient Greek city-state of Sparta, in about 1000 B.C., it was hoped that male lovers would be in the same army regiment. People thought that if a warrior was in the same regiment as his lover, he would fight harder in order to impress him. The Spartan army was one of the most powerful and feared armies in ancient Greece.

A person who is bisexual is someone who is sexually attracted to people of the opposite sex and sexually attracted to people of the same sex. Someone who is bisexual is attracted to, may fall in love with, and may have a sexual relationship with both males and females. *Bi* means *two* and is also the ancient Greek word for *two*.

There have been gay and bisexual relationships all through history, even before ancient Greece. How people feel and think about homosexuality and bisexuality has a lot to do with the culture and the times in which they live.

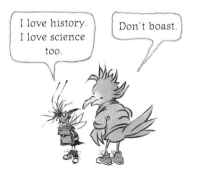

I love history. I love science too.

Don't boast.

Scientists do not completely understand or agree on why one person is straight, why another person is gay, or why another person is bisexual. In fact, there may be more than one reason.

But most scientists believe that being gay, or straight, or bisexual is not something you choose – just as you cannot choose what skin colour you were born with or whether you were born male or female. They believe that a person is born with traits – with the biological make-up – that make him or her develop into a straight person, or gay person, or bisexual person.

Sometimes as children are growing up, boys become curious about other boys, and girls become curious about

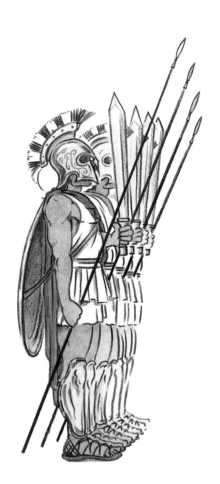

other girls. They may even look at and even touch each other's bodies. This is a normal kind of exploring and does not have anything to do with whether a girl or boy is or will be straight, gay, lesbian or bisexual.

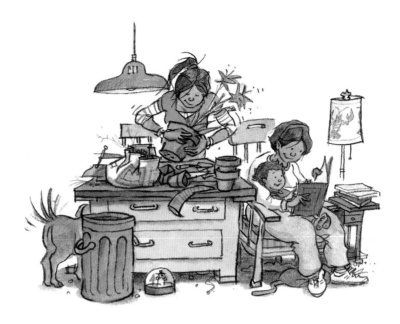

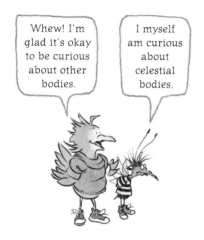

Whew! I'm glad it's okay to be curious about other bodies.

I myself am curious about celestial bodies.

Dreaming about or having a crush on a person of the same sex also does not necessarily mean that a girl or a boy is or will be straight, gay, or lesbian or bisexual.

Many people use the term LGBT. These initials – *L* for *lesbian*, *G* for *gay*, *B* for *bisexual* and *T* for *transgender* – are a way of referring to people who are lesbian, gay, bisexual or transgender.

Transgender is a word that has to do with gender. *Trans* is the Latin word for *across*. *Gender* is another word for whether a person is a female or a male. *Gender* is also about

the thoughts and feelings a person has about being a female or being a male. A *transgender person* is someone who crosses from the gender that person was born with to the opposite gender, or as some say, to the other gender.

This means that a person who was born with a male body, but feels, acts, and knows he is a female – or a person who was born with a female body, but feels, acts, and knows she is a male – is a transgender person. Some may feel this way all of the time and will feel this way throughout their lives. Others may feel this way for only a few months or a few years. And some may feel that sometimes they are one

gender and other times they are the other gender.

People who feel this way may change the way they dress or their name to reflect the gender they believe they really are. They may also ask to be called "he" instead of "she" or "she" instead of "he". Transgender people can be straight, or lesbian, or gay or bisexual.

There are some who disapprove of people who are gay, lesbian, bisexual or transgender or call them offensive names, or tease, bully or even hate them, or don't want to be with them, only because a person is lesbian, gay, bisexual or transgender. Some also feel that LGBT people should not

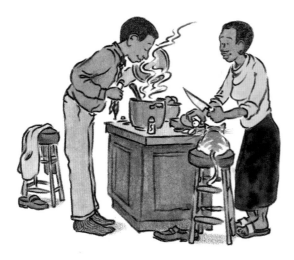
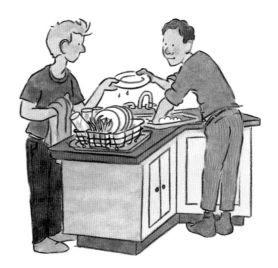

have the right to marry. They may feel this way because they think LGBT people are different from them or that gay relationships are wrong. These people's views are based on fears or misinformation, not on facts. People are often afraid of people they know little or nothing about or who are different from them in some ways.

If a person has any questions, thoughts or concerns about his or her sexual feelings or gender, talking to someone you know and trust – a parent, relative, therapist, doctor, nurse, teacher or clergy member – can be helpful.

No matter what some people may think, it's always important for every person to remember to treat all people with respect. And it's important to know that a person's daily life – making a home, having friends and fun, working, being in love, being single, being a partner, being married, raising children – is mostly the same whether he or she is straight, gay, bisexual or transgender.

PART TWO

Our Bodies

6
The Human Body
All Kinds of Bodies

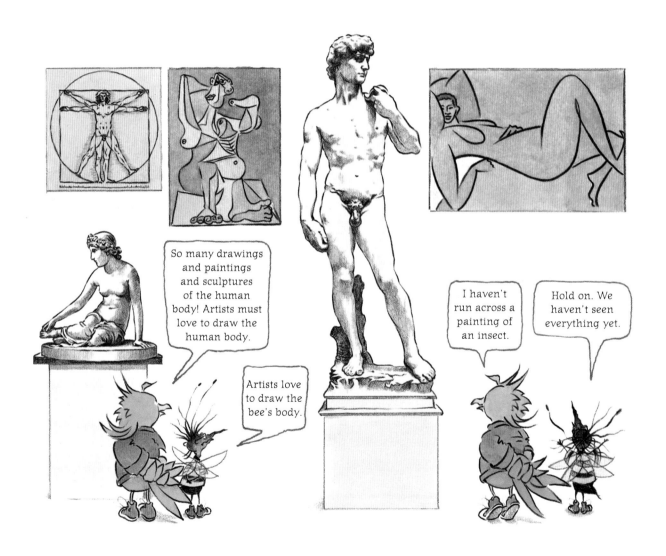

So many drawings and paintings and sculptures of the human body! Artists must love to draw the human body.

Artists love to draw the bee's body.

I haven't run across a painting of an insect.

Hold on. We haven't seen everything yet.

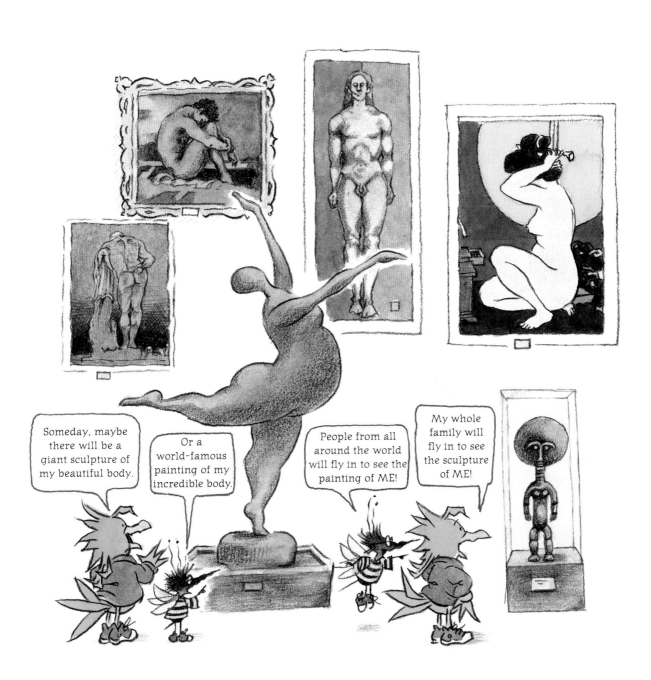

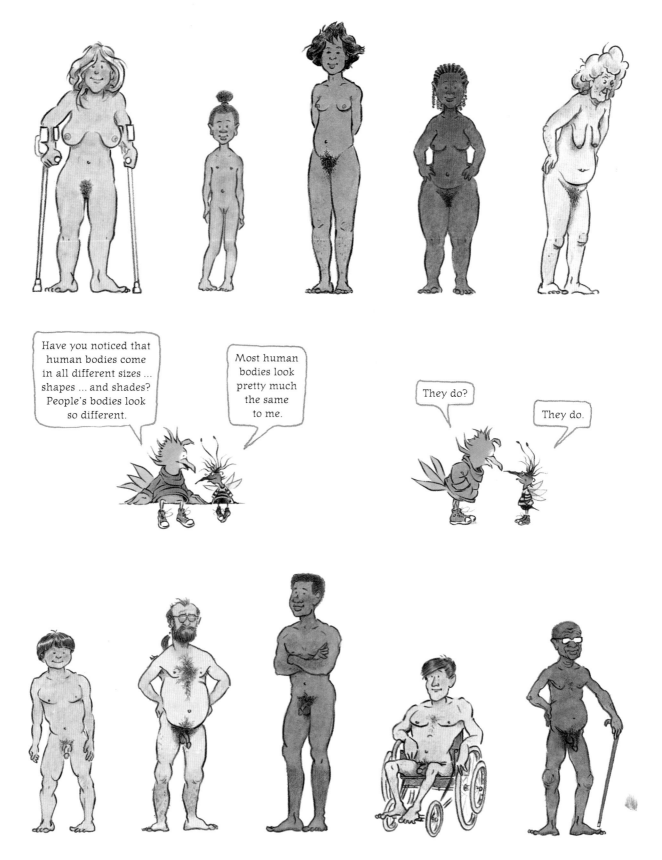

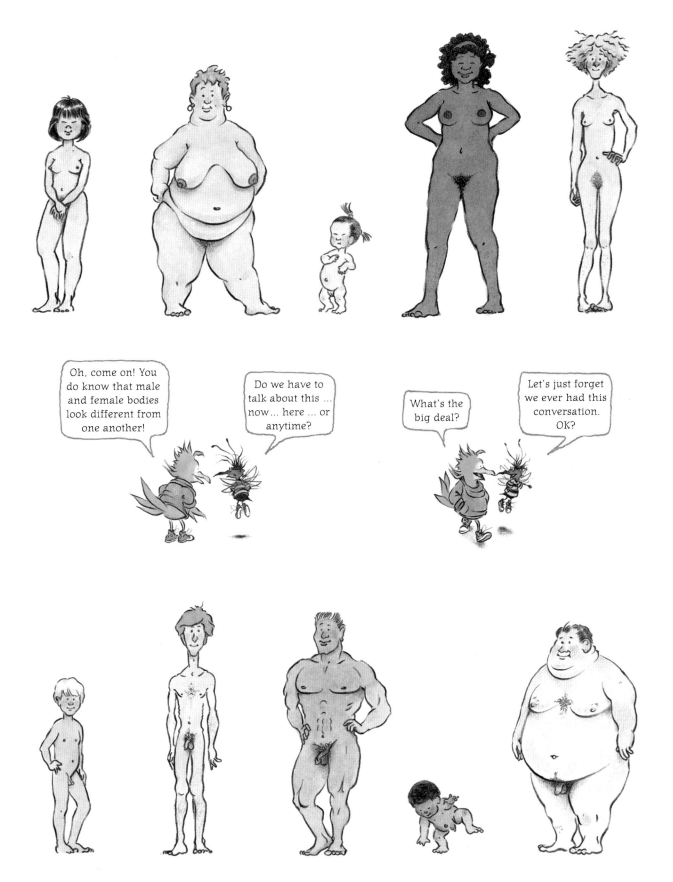

7
Outside and Inside
The Female Sex Organs

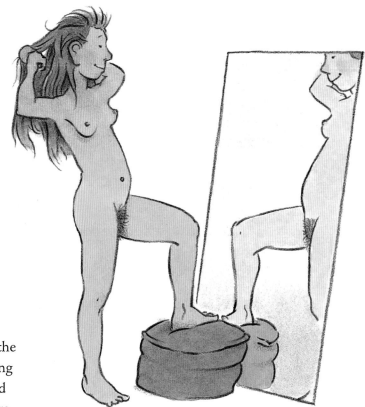

Some of a female's outer sex organs, the clitoris and the opening to the vagina, are hard to see because they are located between her legs.

The Vulva

The whole area of soft skin between a female's legs is called the vulva. The word *vulva* comes from the Latin word *volva,* which means *covering.* The vulva covers the clitoris, the opening to the vagina, the opening to the urethra and the labia.

The Labia

The labia are two sets of soft folds of skin inside the vulva. They cover the inner parts of the vulva – the clitoris, the opening to the urethra, and the opening to the vagina. *Labia* is the Latin word for *lips.*

The Clitoris

The clitoris is a small mound of skin about the size of a pea. When the clitoris is touched and rubbed, a female's body feels good both outside and inside. It feels sort of tingly, sort of warm and nice. It feels sexy.

The Opening to the Urethra

The opening to the urethra is quite small. The urethra is not one of the female's sex organs. It is a tube through which urine – liquid waste – leaves the body.

> BODY FACT: Urine is liquid waste from the body, liquid left over from food and drink that is not used by the body. Urine is the only fluid that travels through a female's urethra.

The Opening to the Vagina

The vagina is a passageway between the uterus – a sex organ inside the female body – and the outside of the female body. The opening to the vagina is bigger than the opening to the urethra.

> BODY FACT: A thin piece of skin, called the hymen, covers part of the opening to the vagina. While a girl is growing – or when she is very active while exercising or playing a sport, or sometimes when she first uses a tampon, or during the first time she has sexual intercourse – the hymen stretches and may tear a bit, and the opening becomes somewhat larger.

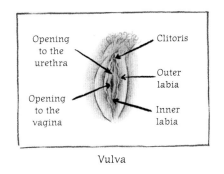

Opening to the urethra — Clitoris

Opening to the vagina — Outer labia

Inner labia

Vulva

The Anus

The anus is a small opening through which faeces – solid waste – leave a female's body.

> BODY FACT: Faeces are the solid material that is left over from food that is not used by the body. They leave the female body in the same way that they leave the male body. Solid waste is stored in the bowel before it leaves the body through the anus.

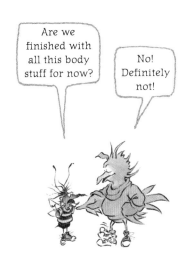

Are we finished with all this body stuff for now?

No! Definitely not!

In all, from front to back, there are three openings between a female's legs: the opening to her urethra, the opening to her vagina, and her anus. If a girl or woman is curious about what these openings look like, she can hold a mirror between her legs and take a look.

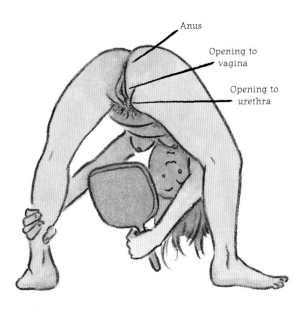

Anus

Opening to vagina

Opening to urethra

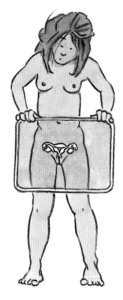

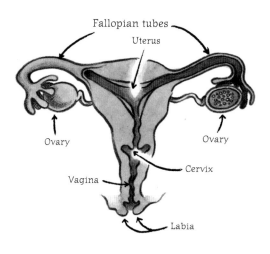

Fallopian tubes

Uterus

Ovary

Ovary

Cervix

Vagina

Labia

If you could actually look inside the female body and see the female's inner sex organs, you would see two ovaries, two Fallopian tubes, the uterus and the vagina.

The Ovaries

The two ovaries – one on each side of the uterus – are about the size of large strawberries. The ovaries contain a female's sex cells – also called eggs or ova. A single egg is called an ovum.

BODY FACT: At birth, a baby girl's ovaries already contain an astonishing number of egg cells – about one to two million. These egg cells are not grown up enough to produce babies until a girl begins to go through puberty. Female puberty – the time when a girl's body starts to grow into a young woman's body – can begin anytime from about the age of eight or nine until fifteen. At puberty, a girl has about three hundred to four hundred thousand egg cells.

A female's egg cells are no longer able to produce babies after the female is about fifty.

Ovaries

The Fallopian Tubes

The two Fallopian tubes are passageways through which an egg travels on its way to the uterus. One end of each tube almost touches an ovary. The other end of each tube is connected to the uterus. Each tube is about three inches long and the width of a drinking straw.

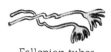

Fallopian tubes

The Uterus

The uterus is made of strong muscles and is hollow inside. It is about the size and shape of a small upside-down pear and is connected to both Fallopian tubes and the inside end of the vagina.

BODY FACT: The uterus is the place in which a developing baby, called a fetus, grows, is fed and is protected. A fetus grows in the uterus, which stretches as the fetus grows bigger, for about nine months until it is ready to be born. The uterus is sometimes called the womb.

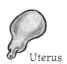

Uterus

The Cervix

The cervix is a small opening located in the lower part of the uterus. It connects the uterus to the top of the vagina. This opening stretches wide when it's time for a baby to be born.

The Vagina

The vagina is the passageway from the uterus to the outside of the female body.

BODY FACT: A baby travels through the vagina when it is ready to be born. The vagina is also the passageway through which a small amount of blood, other fluids and tissue leave the uterus, about once a month. This small amount of normal bleeding is called menstruation or "having a period" and begins when a girl has reached puberty. The vagina is also the place where the penis fits during sexual intercourse.

8
Outside and Inside
The Male Sex Organs

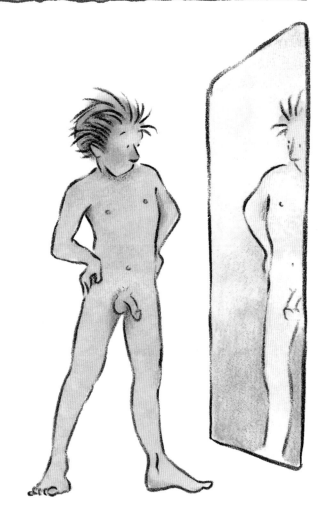

A male's outer sex organs, the penis and the scrotum – which contains the two testicles – are easy to see when a boy or man is naked because they hang between his legs.

The Penis

The penis is made of soft, spongy tissue and blood vessels. Urine – liquid waste – leaves a male's body through a small opening at the tip of his penis.

The end of the penis is called the glans. When the penis is touched and rubbed, a male's body feels good both outside and inside – sort of tingly, sort of warm and nice. It feels sexy.

BODY FACT: Generally, the penis is soft and hangs down over the scrotum. Sometimes, it becomes stiff and hard, and larger and longer, and stands out from the body. This is called an erection.

All males are born with some loose skin covering the end of the penis, called the foreskin. Some male babies have their foreskins removed a few days after they are born, by a doctor or a specially trained religious person. This is called circumcision. Although a circumcised penis looks different from an uncircumcised penis, both work in the same way and equally well.

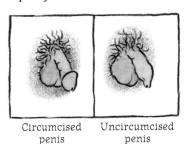

Circumcised   Uncircumcised
penis   penis

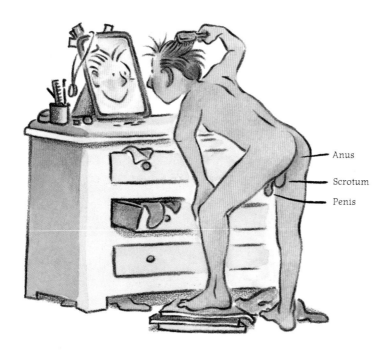

Anus

Scrotum

Penis

The Testicles

The two testicles are soft and squishy and are covered and protected by the scrotum. Usually one testicle hangs lower than the other. Before puberty each testicle is about the size of a marble. During puberty, each testicle grows to about the size of a walnut or a very small ball. That's why they are often called "nuts" or "balls".

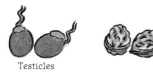

Testicles

BODY FACT: A male's sex cells are produced in the testicles. Unlike female sex cells, which exist at birth, male sex cells are not made until a boy begins to go through puberty. Male puberty – the time when a boy's body starts to grow into a young man's body – can begin anytime from about the age of ten to about fifteen. At that time, a boy begins to produce sex cells. Male sex cells are called sperm, and males continue to make them into old age.

The Scrotum

The scrotum is the soft sac of wrinkly skin that covers, holds and protects the two plum-shaped testicles.

The Anus

The anus is a small opening through which faeces – solid waste – leave a male's body.

BODY FACT: Solid waste is the solid material left over from food that is not used by the body. It leaves the male body in the same way that it leaves the female body – through the anus. Solid waste is stored in the bowel before it leaves the body through the anus.

In all, from front to back, there are two openings between a male's legs: the small opening at the tip of his penis and his anus.

If you could actually look inside the male body and see the male's inner sex organs, you would see two testicles and a series of tubes and glands that are connected to each other.

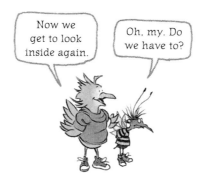

Now we get to look inside again.

Oh, my. Do we have to?

The Epididymis

Each testicle is connected to its own small tube-like structure called the epididymis. Sperm travel through and "grow up" in the epididymis on their way to the vas deferens. Each epididymis is shaped like headphones but is much smaller.

BODY FACT: Each epididymis is a tightly coiled thin tube, which, if stretched out, would be about twenty feet long.

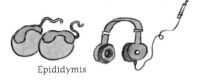

Epididymis

The Vas Deferens

The two vas deferens are each about a foot and a half long. Each of these long, narrow, flexible, and fairly straight tubes starts at the epididymis and winds all the way to the urethra. The two vas deferens are about as flexible as strands of cooked spaghetti.

BODY FACT: Sperm cells travel from each testicle through the epididymis and the vas deferens.

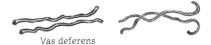

Vas deferens

The Seminal Vesicles and the Prostate Gland

The two seminal vesicles and the prostate gland produce fluids that combine with the sperm to form a mixture called semen. *Semen* is the Latin word for *seed*. The sperm then travel along in the fluids to and through the urethra.

The Urethra

The urethra is a long, narrow tube that carries urine – liquid waste – from the bladder, where it is stored, to the penis and out through the opening at its tip. It is also the passageway through which semen leaves the male body.

BODY FACT: Urine is liquid waste from the body, liquid left over from the food and drink that is not used by the body.

BODY FACT: Semen, which carries a male's sperm, leaves a male's body in rapid spurts through the tip of his penis. This spurting is called ejaculation, and it occurs only after puberty has begun. Both semen and urine come out of the same opening at the tip of the penis. When a male ejaculates, muscles tighten and keep urine in his bladder so that urine does not leave the penis at the same time as semen.

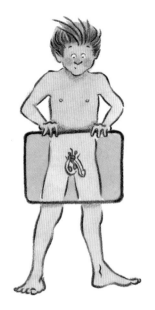

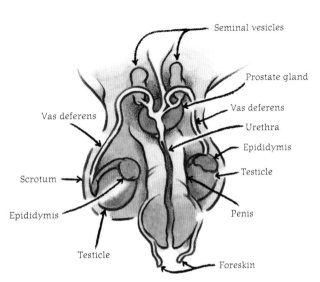

Seminal vesicles

Prostate gland

Vas deferens

Urethra

Epididymis

Testicle

Penis

Foreskin

Vas deferens

Scrotum

Epididymis

Testicle

9
Words
Talking about Bodies and Sex

Children, teenagers and adults use all kinds of words for parts of the body and for sex. Some are scientific words. Some are unscientific – the common, everyday words that people use to talk about bodies and sex. Some of these words are nice, some are funny and some are rude.

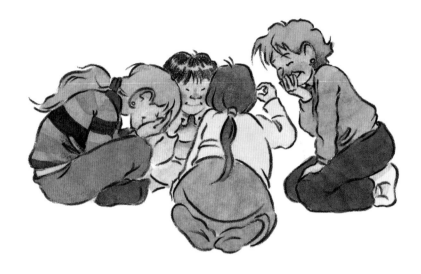

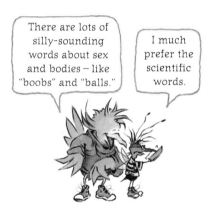

> There are lots of silly-sounding words about sex and bodies – like "boobs" and "balls."

> I much prefer the scientific words.

Everyday words are often called slang words. Rude and disrespectful words about sex and parts of the body are often called "dirty words". Jokes about bodies and sex are some-times called "dirty jokes".

Some people think it's fun to use slang or dirty words and to joke about bodies and sex. Others feel embarrassed or uncomfortable when they hear these words. It's important to respect people's feelings about slang, dirty words or dirty jokes, whatever those feelings may be.

Perhaps people feel uncom-fortable talking about sex and bodies because we do not see our sexual body parts as much as we see our arms, legs, fingers, toes, ears, eyes and noses. After all, our sexual body parts are usually covered by clothes.

Some people think it's wrong to think and talk or joke about bodies and sex. But many people think it can be com-forting and helpful to talk or even joke about sex and bodies with someone you know and trust like a friend, a parent, an older brother or sister, or a cousin.

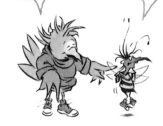

> Did you ever notice that some grown-ups – not just children – have a hard time talking about sex?

> Yep! They twist around in their chairs and say "Well, uh..." about a hundred times or laugh nervously.

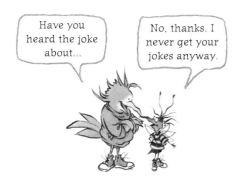

The Joke

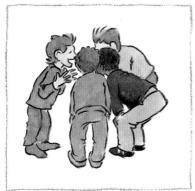 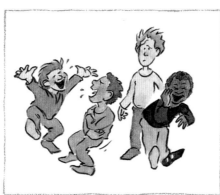 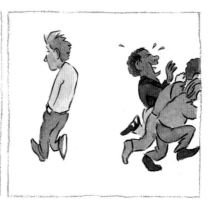

If you don't "get" the joke, you can always ask someone to explain it to you.

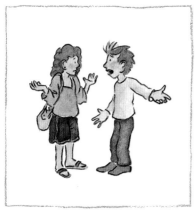 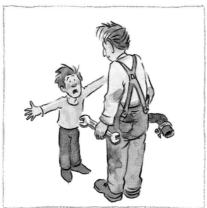 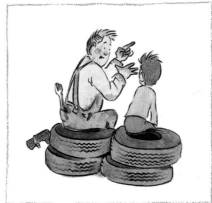

PART THREE

Puberty

10
Changes and Messages
Puberty and Hormones

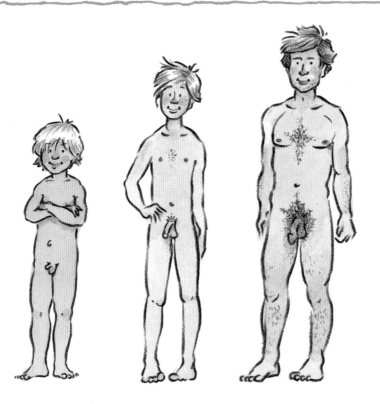

Our bodies change from the moment we are born and keep on changing all through our lives. They change because everything that's alive grows and changes.

There is a time when girls and boys do more than just grow taller and bigger as they have done since birth. Girls start to grow into young women sometime between the ages of eight or nine and fifteen. Boys start to grow into young men sometime between the ages of nine or ten and fifteen.

Puberty is one of the names given to this span of time. The word *puberty* comes from the Latin word *pubertas*, which means *grown-up* or *adult*. When people use the word *puberty*, they are usually talking about all the physical changes that take place in the body during this time. Most of these changes make it physically possible for a female and a male to make a baby.

The other word that is used to describe the span of time between childhood and adulthood is *adolescence*. The word *adolescence* comes from the Latin word *adolescere*, which means to *grow up*. When people use the word *adolescence*, they are usually talking not only about the physical changes that take place during puberty, but also about all the new thoughts, feelings, relationships and responsibilities children have as they become young adults.

Even though the words *adolescence* and *puberty* have somewhat different meanings, people often use them interchangeably.

Puberty, or adolescence, is an in-between time – when a boy or girl is not a child anymore but is not yet an adult.

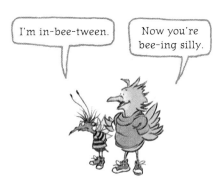

I'm in-bee-tween.

Now you're bee-ing silly.

Girls often start puberty when they are nine or ten or eleven years old. Boys often start puberty a year or so later – when they are ten or eleven or twelve. For most young people, puberty takes place over a stretch of time – over a few years. This usually gives children time to get used to their adult bodies.

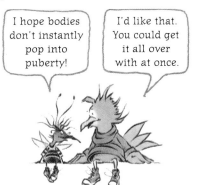

I hope bodies don't instantly pop into puberty!

I'd like that. You could get it all over with at once.

The many changes that take place in our bodies during puberty are caused by hormones. Hormones are chemicals that are produced in many different places in our bodies. Hormones travel through the body's bloodstream from the place where they are made to other places in the body where they do their work.

The word *hormone* comes from the Greek word *hormon*, meaning *to set in motion* – to start something working. There are many kinds of hormones in our bodies.

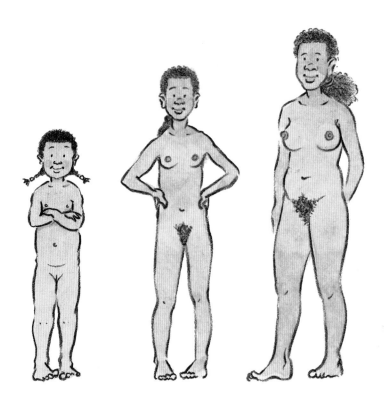

During puberty, the brain begins to manufacture special hormones. These hormones send a message to the sex organs – a boy's testicles or a girl's ovaries – that tells them to start working – to start producing sex hormones.

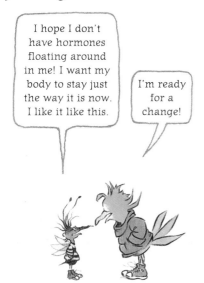

> I hope I don't have hormones floating around in me! I want my body to stay just the way it is now. I like it like this.

> I'm ready for a change!

The sex hormones in the male body then instruct the testicles to make sperm. The sex hormones in the female body then instruct the ovaries to send out an egg.

It is the sex hormones that cause the changes that make children's bodies grow into adult bodies. Only then is it possible for humans to have babies. Once the sex hormones start working, puberty begins.

Some sex hormones cause changes to take place in and around boys' and girls' sex organs. Others cause changes to take place throughout their bodies. Sex hormones can also affect girls' and boys' feelings and moods.

Many cultures, religions, communities and families mark the beginning of puberty for a boy or girl with a celebration or ceremony. They view puberty as a special part of growing up. Others choose to let a boy or girl enter puberty without a celebration or ceremony. They view puberty simply as a regular and ordinary part of growing up.

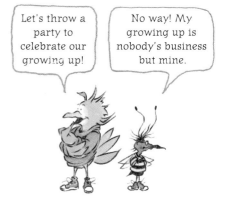

> Let's throw a party to celebrate our growing up!

> No way! My growing up is nobody's business but mine.

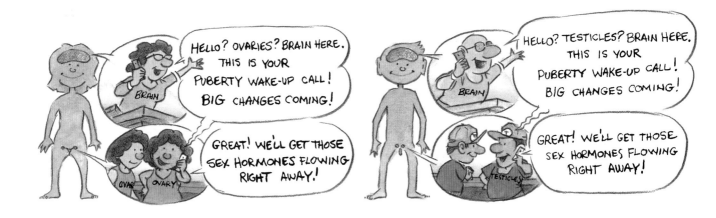

11
The Travels of the Egg
Female Puberty

"Start making female sex hormones!" is one of the messages the female's brain sends to her ovaries at puberty. And the ovaries do just that. They begin to produce the hormones oestrogen and progesterone. Oestrogen tells the eggs, which have been in a girl's ovaries since birth, to grow up. Usually only one egg grows up at a time.

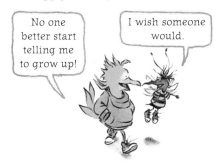

No one better start telling me to grow up!

I wish someone would.

When the eggs grow up, the ovaries do something they've never done before. About once a month, they release a single grown-up egg. An egg is about the size of a grain of sand.

Eggs are female sex cells. A girl's ovaries usually begin releasing eggs during puberty. In her life, she will release about four hundred to five hundred eggs. The release of an egg is called ovulation. The word *ovulation* comes from the Latin word *ovum*, meaning *egg*.

At about the same time every month, when an egg is released from one of the ovaries, it is swept by tiny fingerlike projections into one of the Fallopian tubes, where it begins its travels to the uterus.

The Fallopian tube is the place where an egg can meet and unite with a sperm. Once an egg has united with a sperm, they become the beginning cell of a baby. The uniting of an egg cell and a sperm cell is called conception or fertilization.

The fertilized egg continues to travel through the Fallopian tube and into the uterus, where the female sex hormone progesterone has helped to create a soft lining that is ready to receive it. The fertilized egg then plants itself in the lining of the uterus. This soft, thick, cosy lining is made of extra blood vessels, tissue and other fluids and is created so that the fertilized egg will have a healthy place to grow.

If the egg has been fertilized, it will usually plant itself in the uterus and stay there – and grow into a baby. However, most of the time, the egg is not fertilized. If the egg does not unite with a sperm within about twenty-four to thirty-six hours after leaving an ovary, it does not stay in the uterus and does not go on to develop into a baby.

Instead, the egg breaks down while it is in the uterus and mixes with some of the extra blood and fluid in the soft lining of the uterus. Since there is no fertilized egg starting to grow in the uterus, this soft lining is not needed and dissolves. It then passes out of the uterus, through the vagina, and out of the body in the form of a small amount of blood, other fluids and tissue. The lining's monthly passing out of the uterus and the vagina is called menstruation. The word *menstruation* comes from the Latin word *mensis*, which means *month*.

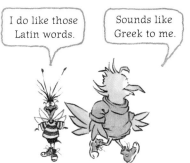

I do like those Latin words.

Sounds like Greek to me.

THE TRAVELS OF THE EGG: *Menstruation*

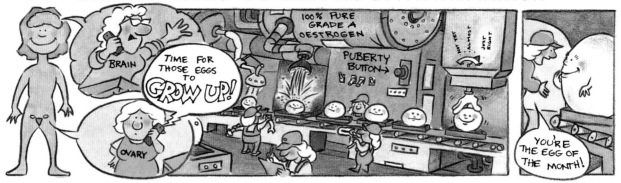

At puberty the brain tells the ovaries to produce oestrogen, which tells the eggs to mature.

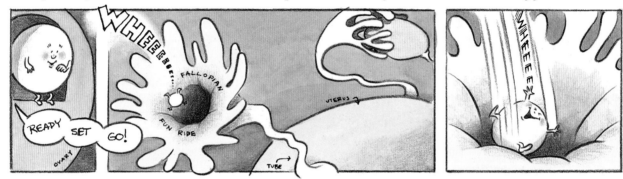

And then, about once a month, an egg leaves an ovary and pops into a Fallopian tube,

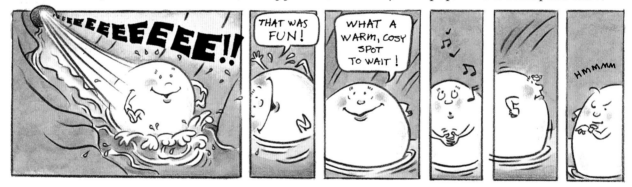

where it waits before travelling to the uterus.

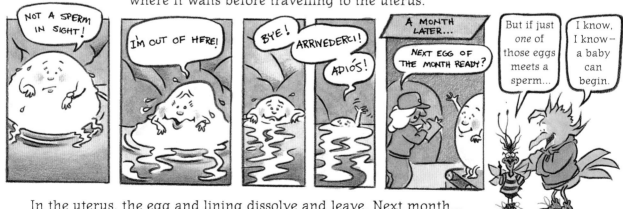

In the uterus, the egg and lining dissolve and leave. Next month...

The period of time from the beginning of one menstruation to the next is about a month long and is called the menstrual cycle.

Girls usually start to menstruate after their ovaries have begun to release eggs. As soon as a girl's ovaries have begun to release eggs, she can become pregnant if she has had sexual intercourse.

But some girls may begin to release eggs even before they start to menstruate. This means that it is possible, although quite rare, for a girl to become pregnant before she has started to menstruate. Girls usually start to menstruate at the age of eleven or twelve. But some start as early as age nine and others start as late as age fifteen, and that's perfectly normal.

The very first time a girl menstruates, she may worry that a large amount of blood will suddenly flow out. In fact, the blood usually comes out slowly. Only a few tablespoonfuls to about half a cup of blood and tissue dribble out during each menstruation. But the amount can be more or less, and that's also perfectly normal.

This dribbling continues over a period of a few days. That's why people call menstruation a menstrual period or "having your period". Other children call menstruation "my friend", "that time of the month", or "the curse". No matter what people call it, menstruation is a healthy occurrence.

A period usually lasts about three to eight days. When a girl first starts to menstruate, her periods often come irregularly – sometimes a few weeks apart, sometimes many weeks apart. It can often take up to one or two years for a girl's period to occur on a regular schedule – about once a month. Some girls' and women's periods never become very regular. If that happens, it's a good idea to check with a nurse or doctor – just to make sure it's normal for you.

Most girls and women continue their regular activities during menstruation. For example, they have baths and showers, swim, play sport, dance and do whatever they normally like to do. Some girls and women do get cramps – usually slight, tight pains around the area of the uterus – before and during their periods. Most cramps are normal.

When girls and women travel, play sport vigorously, lose or gain a lot of weight, or become upset or ill, their periods can become irregular for a while. And when a female becomes pregnant, her periods stop until after the baby is born.

When women are about fifty years old, their bodies start to make fewer sex hormones. As a result, their ovaries stop releasing eggs, and they stop menstruating. This period of time in a woman's life is called menopause – the pausing and stopping of menstruation. When a woman stops having menstrual periods, she is no longer able to become pregnant.

During a menstrual period, a girl or woman uses sanitary towels or tampons to absorb the menstrual flow that passes out of her vagina so it will not leak on her knickers or other clothes. She can use whichever is more comfortable.

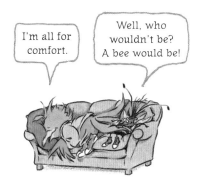

Sanitary towels are also called pads. *Sanitary* means *clean.*

Where a Towel Fits

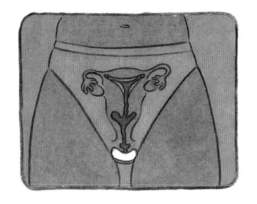

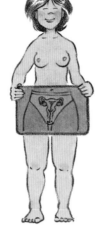

Where a Tampon Fits

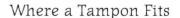

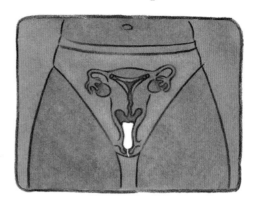

Towels

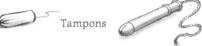

Tampons

Towels and tampons are made of a clean, soft, cottonlike material and absorb the menstrual flow. A towel fits on the inside of a girl or woman's knickers, just outside the opening to her vagina. Most towels come with a small piece of adhesive tape on one side that keeps them in place.

Tampons fit inside the vagina. A tampon cannot move into the uterus because the cervix is too small an opening for a tampon to pass through.

One way a girl can find out when she might get her first period is to ask her mother. If her mother started menstruating early, there's a good chance she may start early too. If her mother started later, there's a good chance that she may start later.

Talking to someone about menstruation – your mother, grandmother or aunt, or an older friend or cousin – can be helpful. A girl can find out many

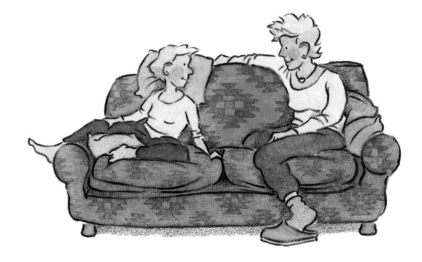

useful things from someone who is already menstruating, such as what it feels like to menstruate, what she will need to do to get ready for her first period, where to get towels or tampons, and how to use them. This kind of information can help prepare a girl for her first period – whether it starts when she is at home or out with friends or in school. She may also want to carry a towel or tampon in her bag in case she gets her first period when she is not at home.

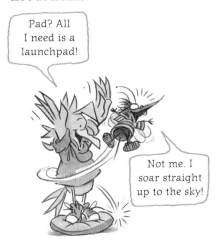

No matter how well prepared she is, a girl's first period usually comes as something of a surprise. For some girls, it may feel quite exciting; for others, a bit scary. But no matter how a girl feels, starting to menstruate is a perfectly normal and natural part of growing up. Most girls feel that starting to menstruate is one of the biggest changes of puberty.

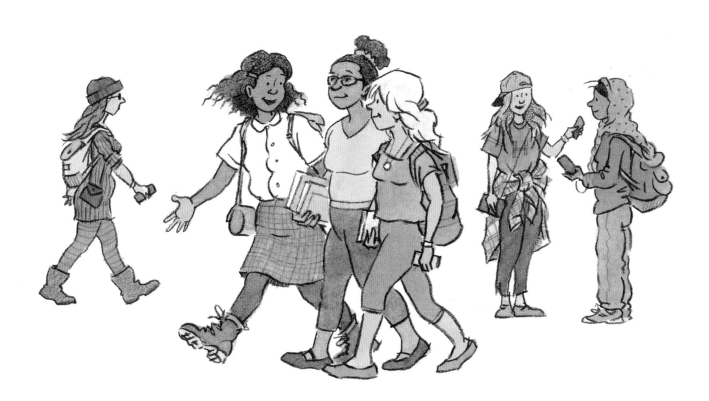

12
The Travels of the Sperm
Male Puberty

"Start making the male sex hormone testosterone!" is one of the messages a boy's brain sends out to his testicles during puberty. And the testicles do just that. They begin to produce testosterone, which causes the male body to grow and change in many new ways.

One of the most important things testosterone does is instruct the testicles to begin to make sperm – something the testicles have never done before.

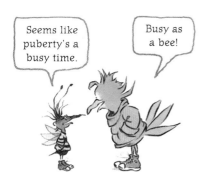

Seems like puberty's a busy time.

Busy as a bee!

Sperm are male sex cells. Unlike girls, boys do not start making sex cells until they reach puberty. Starting at puberty, however, the testicles make a phenomenal number of sperm – about one hundred million to three hundred million sperm per day. That's anywhere from

about one thousand to three thousand sperm every second.

The scrotum protects the testicles by keeping them at the right temperature to make sperm, not too cold and not too hot, just a few degrees below the body's temperature. If it is too cold, the scrotum pulls up the testicles closer to the body to keep them warm enough to make sperm. When a man or boy is swimming in cold water, he can often feel his scrotum tighten as it pulls up his testicles. If it is too hot, the scrotum hangs down loosely, away from the body, again keeping the testicles at just the right temperature to make sperm.

After sperm are produced, the sperm from the right testicle travel through the right epididymis, and the sperm from the left testicle travel through the left epididymis. As they travel, the sperm grow up enough to be able to fertilize – to unite with – a female's egg.

Sperm travel through the vas deferens and pass by the seminal vesicles. As sperm pass by, they mix with fluid from

the seminal vesicles and the prostate gland.

The mixture of sperm and fluid is now called semen. Semen is sticky, cloudy, and whitish. Chemicals in it keep the sperm healthy as they travel into the urethra, through it, and out the tip of the penis. Sperm leave the male body when a male ejaculates semen. *To ejaculate* means *to suddenly release* or *to let go*. When a male ejaculates, his penis is usually erect.

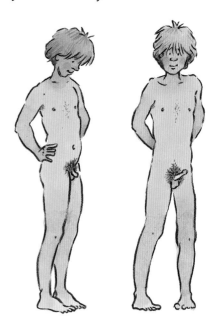

Here's what happens inside a male's body when he has an erection: When his penis is not

THE TRAVELS OF THE SPERM: *Ejaculation*

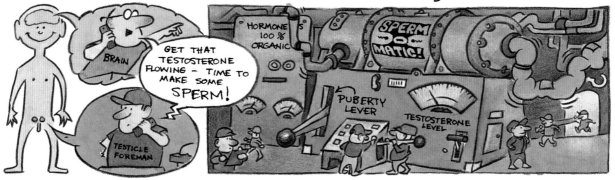

At puberty the brain tells the testicles to produce testosterone and sperm.

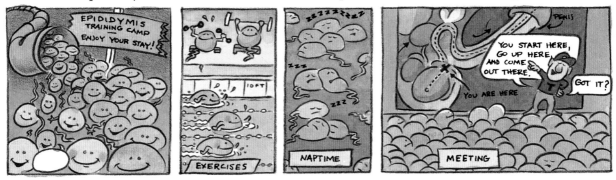

Sperm travel to the epididymis, where they mature and travel

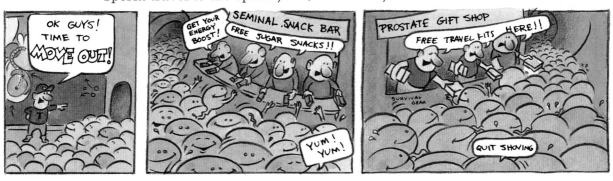

through the vas deferens, past the seminal vesicles and prostate gland,

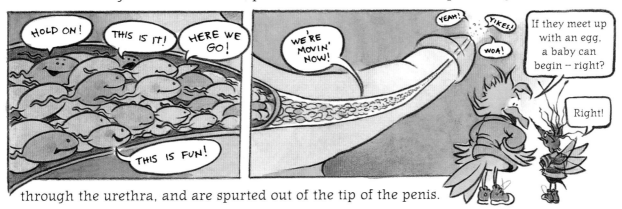

through the urethra, and are spurted out of the tip of the penis.

erect, blood trickles in and out of the penis continuously. But when he has an erection, the muscles that allow blood to flow in and out of his penis open wide and allow more blood to be pumped in, while other muscles tighten and keep the extra amount of blood from leaving the penis. This causes the spongy tissue inside the penis to fill up, which in turn makes the penis become stiff, erect and stand out from the body. This filling up is called an erection.

When the erection is over, the muscles relax and allow the blood to flow back out of the penis and into the body again. And the penis becomes soft again.

A male can have an erection when his penis is touched and rubbed; when he has pleasurable thoughts or sees someone who makes him feel happy, excited, sexy or nervous; when he is watching a film or television programme or video or reads or sees something online that excites him; when someone attractive to him walks by; or when he is having a pleasurable dream.

Males often have erections when they wake up. If a male's bladder – the place where urine is stored in his body – is full, the full bladder excites some nerves at the base of his penis,

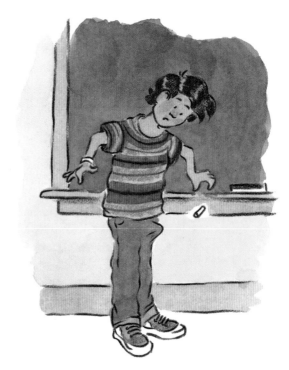

which causes more blood to flow into the penis. This kind of erection has little to do with sexy thoughts and feelings.

Males usually have erections before and during sexual intercourse. An erection makes it possible for the penis to enter the vagina. Sometimes males have erections for no apparent reason, even when they don't want to have them.

Some people call an erection a "hard-on" or "boner" even though there are no bones in the penis. Erections usually last a few seconds, to a few minutes, to half an hour, or more. Males can have erections from the time they are little babies until they are old men – even while they sleep.

Here's what happens inside a male's body when he has an ejaculation: muscles in each epididymis, in each vas deferens, and in the seminal vesicles, along with muscles around the prostate gland, tighten and push the semen into the urethra. The semen, which contains sperm, travels through the urethra and spurts out through the tip of the penis. This spurting out of semen – ejaculation – causes a feeling of excitement called an orgasm.

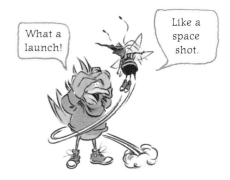

What a launch!

Like a space shot.

During ejaculation, muscles tighten so that urine does not leave the penis at the same time as semen. After ejaculation, the penis becomes soft again and is no longer erect.

There are usually about two to five hundred million sperm spurted out in a single ejaculation – about a teaspoonful of semen. Males can and do have erections without ejaculating any semen. When this happens, the blood leaves the penis slowly and returns to the body's bloodstream, the erection slowly goes away, and the penis becomes soft again and hangs down as usual. It is possible, although this does not happen often, for a male to ejaculate without having an erection.

Boys start to be able to ejaculate during puberty and continue into old age. Ejaculation usually occurs during sexual intercourse. It can also occur during other kinds of sexual touching and excitement and even during sleep.

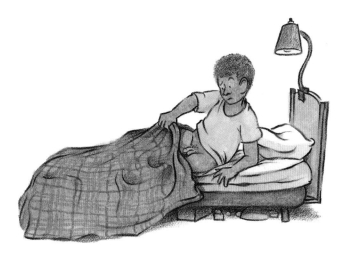

Boys usually start having "wet dreams" at puberty. Wet dreams occur during sleep when a boy is having a pleasurable, exciting or sexy dream and ejaculates some semen. When the boy wakes up, his pyjamas or sheets may be wet and sticky from the ejaculated semen.

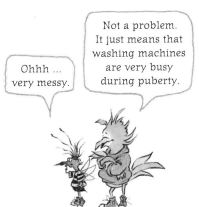

Ohhh ... very messy.

Not a problem. It just means that washing machines are very busy during puberty.

The scientific term for a wet dream is *nocturnal emission*. *Nocturnal* means *occurring at night*. *Emission* means *a release, a letting go*. Wet dreams are usual and normal events for boys. A boy's first ejaculation often happens during a dream.

Once a male has begun to produce sperm, if just one of his sperm unites with an egg during sexual intercourse, the female can become pregnant and the united cell can grow and develop into a baby.

Many boys feel that starting to ejaculate is one of the biggest changes of puberty.

13
Not All at Once!
Growing and Changing Bodies

During puberty, the sex hormones cause boys and girls to grow and change in even more ways.

All these changes do not take place at once. Most of them happen slowly over a few years' time; a few happen quickly. And they often, although not always, take place in a fairly specific order.

Girls: Puberty Changes
• Ovaries gradually grow larger.
• Body sweats more.
• Skin and hair become more oily.
• Body has a sudden growth spurt.
• Body gains some weight and grows taller.
• Arms and legs grow longer.
• Hands and feet grow bigger.
• Bones in the face grow larger and longer, and the face looks less childlike.
• Soft, darkish hair grows around the vulva and later becomes curly, thick and coarse.
• A tiny bit of sticky, whitish fluid may come out of the vagina.

PUBERTY FACT: The whitish fluid that may flow out of the vagina is normal and helps keep it clean and healthy.

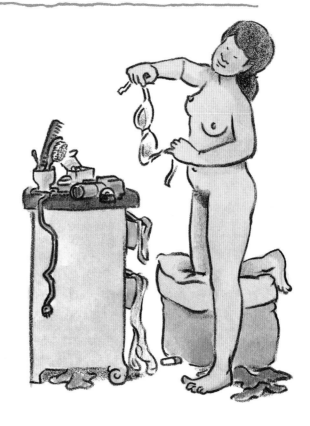

• Hips grow wider. Body begins to look more curvy.

PUBERTY FACT: A girl's hips grow wider, so that if and when she decides to have a baby, her baby will have enough room to leave the uterus when it is ready to be born.

• Hair grows under the arms.
• Breasts and nipples gradually grow larger and fuller.

PUBERTY FACT: A girl's breasts grow larger and fuller to prepare her body to make milk to nurse her baby if and when she has one.

• Nipples may become a darker colour.
• Menstruation can begin.

PUBERTY FACT: Once the ovaries have grown larger, they start to release mature eggs, and menstruation begins. Once menstruation starts, a girl can become pregnant.

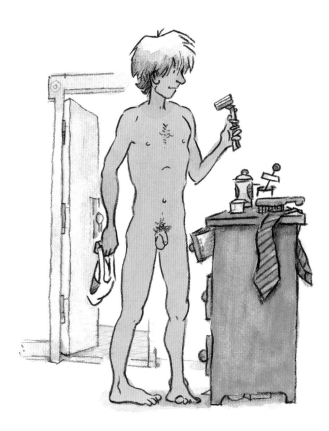

Boys: Puberty Changes

- Testicles gradually grow larger and fuller.
- Penis gradually grows larger and longer.
- Body sweats more.
- Skin and hair become more oily.
- Body has a sudden growth spurt.
- Body gains weight and grows taller.
- Arms and legs grow longer.
- Hands and feet grow larger.
- Bones in the face grow, and the face looks less childlike.
- Soft, darkish hair grows around the base of the penis and later becomes curly, thick and coarse.

- Hair grows under the arms.
- Shoulders and chest grow bigger.
- Bigger muscles develop.
- Scrotum turns a darker colour.
- Hair grows on the face, first the moustache, then the beard and sideburns.
- Hair grows on the chest.

> PUBERTY FACT: Sometimes the area around a boy's nipples may feel sore and may even swell. This is caused by the hormones that are released during puberty. The soreness and swelling go away after a few months.

- The larynx, or as it is commonly called, the voice box, grows bigger.

- The voice cracks and then becomes deeper.
- The Adam's apple may begin to show more.

> PUBERTY FACT: When a boy's voice begins to change, one second it can sound high, one second low, and the next high again, causing a cracking-squeaky sound. But after a while, a boy's voice begins to sound deeper and lower, because the larynx and vocal cords have grown. As the larynx grows bigger, it may push the Adam's apple forward, causing it to show more.

- Sperm begin to be produced.
- Ejaculations – including wet dreams – begin to occur.

> PUBERTY FACT: Once a male can make sperm, if he has intercourse and if the female's ovaries have started to release eggs, she can become pregnant.

At this age, young people's bodies change more dramatically and rapidly than at any other time in their lives – except for the very first year of life.

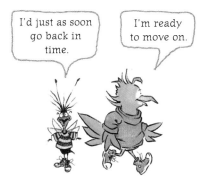

I'd just as soon go back in time.

I'm ready to move on.

14
More Changes!
Taking Care of Your Body

Many of the physical changes that take place during puberty cause our bodies to work in many new ways. This means that young people have to learn some new ways to take care of their bodies.

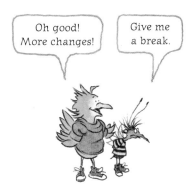

Oh good! More changes!

Give me a break.

Girls and boys grow more hair during puberty. They grow hair under their arms. The hair on their arms and legs grows thicker and longer – especially boys' hair.

Hair called pubic hair also grows – for a girl around her vulva, and for a boy around the base of his penis – directly in front of a bone called the pubic bone.

The amount of hair that grows on boys' faces, chests, arms and legs during puberty varies greatly, from hardly any to a lot.

Some boys and girls start shaving during puberty. For most, shaving is a choice. Some females choose to shave the hair that grows under their arms and on their legs, and some don't. Some males choose to shave their beards and moustaches, and some don't. However, some religious groups require that their boys and men not use a razor or scissors to cut their hair.

During puberty, a person's sweat glands produce more sweat than before. Both boys and girls start to sweat under their arms and develop a new kind of body odour, sometimes from under their arms, sometimes from their feet, and sometimes from all over their bodies.

That's one of the reasons children going through puberty have a lot of baths or showers and wash their bodies and hair a lot. This new kind of sweating is often one of the first signs that puberty is starting. Washing with soap and using a deodorant can help get rid of most strong body odours.

Some young people sweat a lot; some a little. It is likely that you will sweat about the same amount as your father or mother did while he or she was going through puberty.

Some young people's hair becomes oily during puberty. Often some oiliness also begins to appear on the nose and forehead.

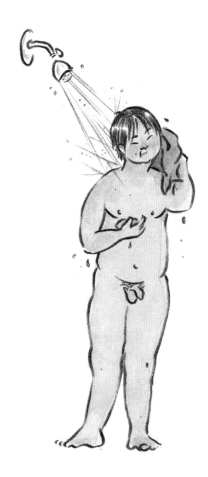

During puberty, most boys and girls develop spots on their faces – mostly on their noses and foreheads. Sometimes, young people develop spots on their backs and chests. Spots are sometimes called "zits".

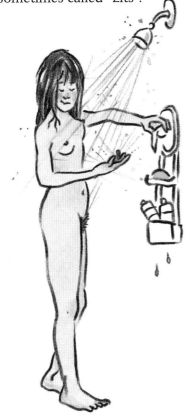

Although careful washing with soap and water is a good way to care for the skin, sometimes it is not enough. Creams and medicines can help control spots. Some can be bought directly from a pharmacy without a written prescription; others need to be prescribed by a doctor and then purchased from a pharmacy or online.

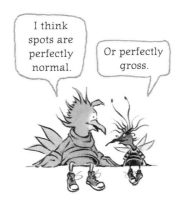

I think spots are perfectly normal.

Or perfectly gross.

Though it's true that no one likes having spots, having them is perfectly normal. Young people develop spots and/or oily hair and sweat more during puberty because their oil and sweat glands are more active than ever before.

Puberty is the time when many girls, if they choose to, start to wear a bra. *Bra* is short for the word *brassière.* A girl often goes with her mother, grandmother, older sister, aunt or a friend to buy her first bra.

It is not necessary to wear a bra to keep breasts healthy. Girls and women who wear bras do so because they feel more comfortable wearing them. Some wear a bra only when they are exercising or playing sport. Others wear one all the time, except when sleeping. Still others never wear a bra at all. No matter what size breasts a girl or woman has, she can buy a bra that fits her. Bras are made with different size cups in order to support various breast sizes.

Many boys and men wear jockstraps when playing sports. A jockstrap fits over the testicles and penis, keeping them in place and protecting them from bruises or injuries. When playing some contact sports such as rugby, hockey or cricket, a male can slip a plastic cup, called an athletic box, into the front of his jockstrap to provide even more protection for his testicles and penis. Athletic cups also come in various sizes.

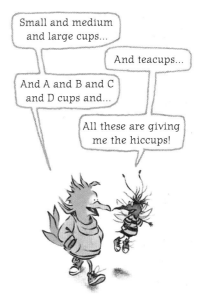

Small and medium and large cups...

And teacups...

And A and B and C and D cups and...

All these are giving me the hiccups!

Girls' and boys' bodies change in so many ways during puberty that taking care of them can at times be a chore. However, eating healthy foods, exercising and keeping fit, keeping clean and getting enough sleep can help a boy or girl feel healthy and good about all the growing and changing that goes on.

15
Back and Forth, Up and Down
New and Changing Feelings

The many changes that take place in young people's bodies during puberty are often accompanied by new and strong feelings about how their bodies look, feel and act – and by new and strong feelings about growing up and sex.

Many young people find these changes exciting and feel great about their bodies. And just as many find these changes overwhelming and feel shy or embarrassed about their changing bodies. Most young people, at one time or another during puberty, feel confused, uncomfortable, and even scared by these big and sometimes rapid changes.

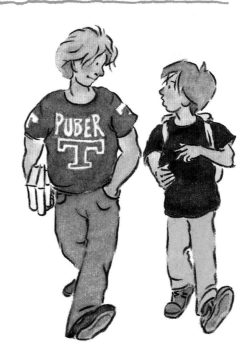

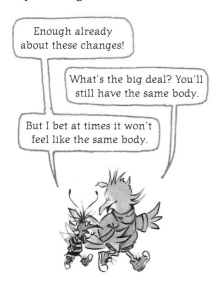

Enough already about these changes!

What's the big deal? You'll still have the same body.

But I bet at times it won't feel like the same body.

Girls and boys often wonder about the size of individual body parts. The truth is – whether small, medium, or large – the size of a person's body parts has nothing to do with how well they work.

It is also true that different bodies develop in different ways. Some girls develop small breasts, others develop medium-sized breasts, and still others develop large breasts. Some boys develop small penises, others develop medium-sized penises, and still others develop large penises. Breasts and penises come in all sorts of sizes.

A girl who develops small breasts may resemble her mother, grandmother or another female relative. And a boy who develops little body hair may resemble his father, grandfather or another male relative. The size of any part of a person's body is mostly inherited from a person's family.

The age when a boy or girl begins puberty is often the same as it was for a close family member of the same sex. You might want to ask your mother, father, or other members of your family what puberty was like for them and when they began to go through it. You might find some clues about how you may develop.

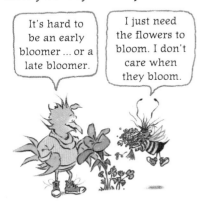

It's hard to be an early bloomer ... or a late bloomer.

I just need the flowers to bloom. I don't care when they bloom.

Girls and boys often wonder whether it matters if their bodies go through puberty slow or fast, early or late, or first or last. When your body changes, or how fast or slowly your body changes, has nothing to

do with how your body will look and perform.

Even so, among one's friends or in one's class, it can be hard to be the first or last girl who menstruates, or the first or last boy whose voice changes; or the first or last girl to wear a bra, or the first or last boy to shave; or the shortest kid one year and the tallest the next year.

Unfortunately, girls and boys tease other children about the ways their bodies look and grow during puberty. A young person's arms, hands, legs and feet may grow longer and bigger before the rest of his or her body catches up. Or a boy's voice may crack right in the middle of a sentence, or a girl may develop a large spot on her forehead just before going to a party. Often these are the kinds of things

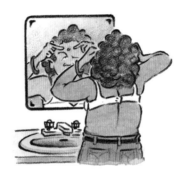

young people are teased about as they go through puberty.

Many young people worry about their friendships during puberty – probably because puberty is a time when some young people start to have boy-friends or girlfriends. One of your friends, even your best friend, may begin to be interested in and sexually attracted to other people, whereas you are not the least bit interested. One of your friends may start to have a boyfriend or girlfriend. Or you may have a boyfriend or girlfriend when your best friend doesn't.

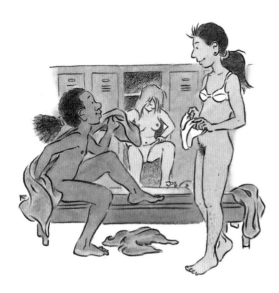

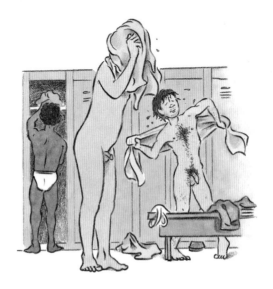

Sometimes young people feel upset or jealous when a friend has a boyfriend or a girlfriend and starts spending time with that person. Although many old friendships stay strong during puberty, some friendships change. Boyfriends and girlfriends are another thing young people are teased about during puberty.

With all the different things that happen to their bodies during puberty, it's no wonder both boys and girls have so many different feelings. They can often feel moody or crabby or even tearful and cry more than usual. And their moods can change quickly. A boy or girl may be laughing at one moment and feel like crying the next.

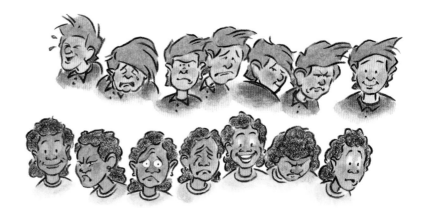

These different feelings often swing back and forth and up and down, like a yo-yo. The increased activity of the sex hormones is one of many factors that causes young people to have mood swings as well as new and strong feelings during puberty.

As girls' and boys' bodies change into grown-up bodies, young people are not always sure that they are ready to be grown-up. Sometimes they want to be treated as children. Other times they want to be treated as adults.

Changing from a child to an adult has its difficult moments. But sooner or later, young people get used to, become comfortable with, and feel good about their more grown-up bodies.

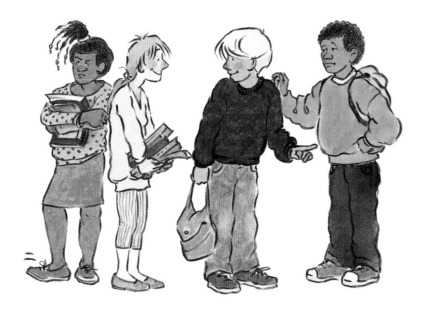

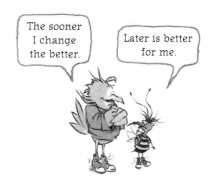

The sooner I change the better.

Later is better for me.

16
Perfectly Normal
Masturbation

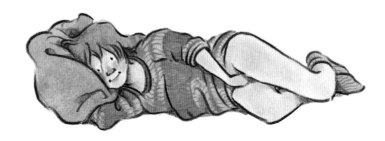

During puberty, when the sex hormones cause boys' and girls' sex organs to become more active, many teenagers begin to have even more pleasurable and excited feelings about their own bodies – and they may also be more attracted to and interested in other people's bodies.

These feelings are often called sexual feelings or "feeling sexy". Even though they are hard to describe, they are normal feelings. They happen at different times and in different ways for different people.

Boys and girls, teenagers, and grown-ups too, experience sexy feelings when they masturbate. Masturbation is touching or rubbing any of your body's sex organs for pleasure – because it feels good. One everyday term for masturbating is "playing with yourself".

Some people think that masturbation is wrong or harmful. And some religions call masturbation a sin. But masturbating cannot hurt you. And it does not result in pregnancy or in getting or passing on infections that are spread by sexual contact.

Many people masturbate. Many don't. Whether you masturbate or not is your choice. Masturbating is perfectly normal.

When people masturbate, they usually rub their sex organs with their hands or with something soft, like a pillow.

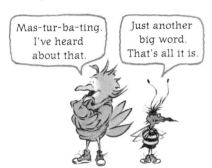

Mas-tur-ba-ting. I've heard about that.

Just another big word. That's all it is.

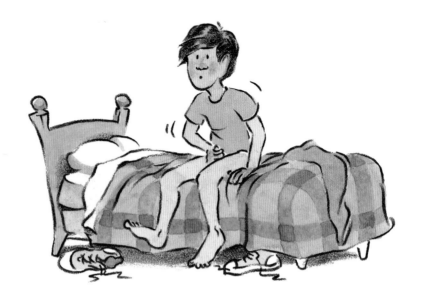

A girl often rubs her clitoris; a boy often rubs his penis. Both the clitoris and the penis are sensitive to touch.

A person may have a warm, good, tingly, exciting feeling all through her or his body while masturbating. This feeling can become more and more intense until it reaches a peak or climax. At that moment, a male may ejaculate; a female may feel strong, exciting sensations just in the area around her vulva or throughout her body. A female may also feel some wetness in her vagina.

For both females and males, this is called having an orgasm.

Some people call it "coming". After having an orgasm, a person usually feels quite content and relaxed.

Usually, but not always, people have orgasms when they masturbate or when they have sexual intercourse. Both boys and girls may also have orgasms during a dream. People may have orgasms at some times and not at other times. Not everyone has orgasms.

Often when people masturbate, they daydream about someone or something happy or pleasurable or sexy. Some people become sexually excited without masturbating, just by looking at sexy pictures or by dreaming about or having fantasies about something pleasurable.

People of all ages masturbate – babies, children, teenagers, grown-ups, and the elderly. Girls and boys often start to masturbate at puberty, but many start before.

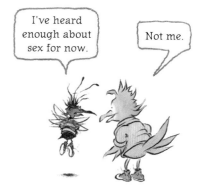

I've heard enough about sex for now.

Not me.

PART FOUR
Families and Babies

17
All Sorts of Families
Caring for Children

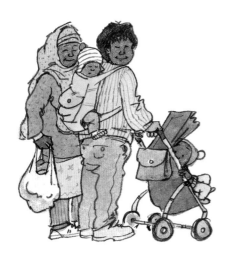

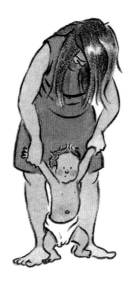

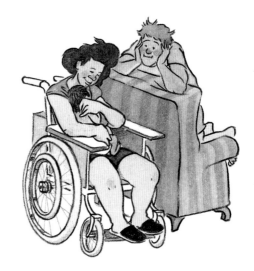

Babies and children grow up in all sorts of families. There are children whose mother and father live together, or whose mother and father live apart, or who have only one parent, or whose parent or parents have adopted them, or who live with a parent and a stepparent, or who live with an aunt, an uncle, a grandmother, a grandfather or other relative, or who have gay or lesbian parents, or who have foster parents.

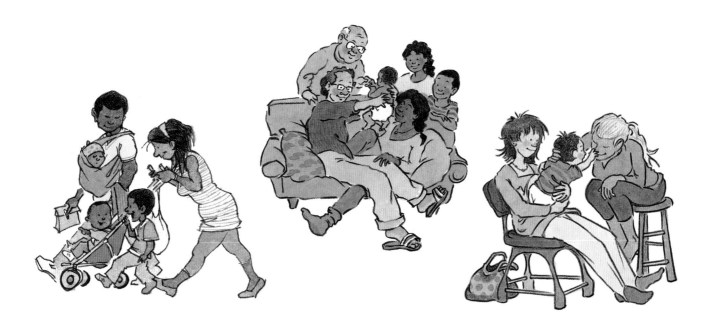

Grandparents and cousins and uncles and aunts are also part of a person's family. And some people feel that their good friends are part of their families too. Most children are loved and taken care of by family members and family friends.

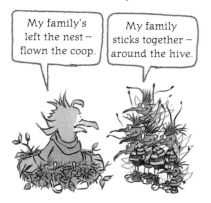

> My family's left the nest – flown the coop.

> My family sticks together – around the hive.

Bringing a baby into this world is an important and exciting event. Becoming a parent is one of the biggest changes that can happen to a person. It brings with it all sorts of new and different responsibilities.

These responsibilities include taking good care of oneself as well as of one's baby and family. That's why the decision about when to start a family is so important. Although it is physically possible for a girl and a boy to make a baby once the girl has started to menstruate (and in rare instances, even before) and once the boy has begun to produce sperm, it makes good sense for people to wait until they are ready and old enough to take on such big responsibilities.

Having a baby when a person is too young can be difficult. There are lots of reasons for this.

Babies of children and young teenagers are often born weighing too little even after a full nine months in the uterus. Babies who weigh too little are more likely to have health problems at birth and as they grow up.

> Babies are pretty cute. Something to love – so soft and cuddly.

> But you don't have to take care of one all day long, all night long, day in, day out, feed the baby, give it a bath, watch it, play with it, get it dressed and undressed, change its nappies...

> I get the picture.

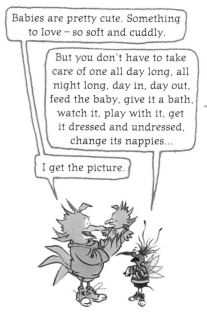

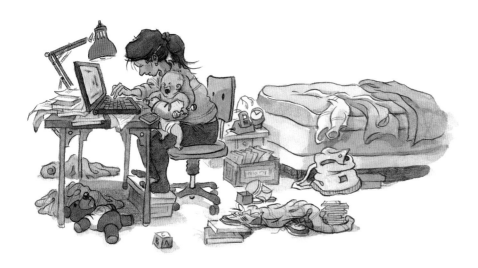

of a baby while they go to school or to work.

Babies are very special and mothers and fathers love their babies a lot, whether a parent is young or old or in between. But it's usually easier and healthier for young people to wait until they are older to have a baby. It gives the baby and the parents a better chance to have a healthy start together.

Parents often find it hard to care for a baby, especially if they are still children or young teenagers. Young people who have a baby often lose the freedom to do what they want to do. It's hard to go out with friends or to get schoolwork done when a baby is around. Babies need a lot of attention, day in, day out, every day, every night.

Teenagers who have babies often drop out of school because they need to work. It costs a lot of money to buy food, clothes, toys and medicine for a baby. It's often hard for teenagers to get a job to pay for these things. And it costs a lot of money to pay someone else to take care

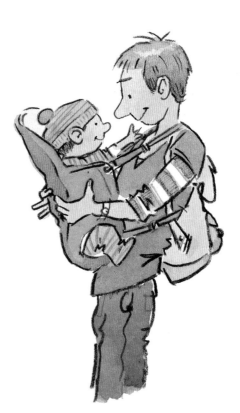

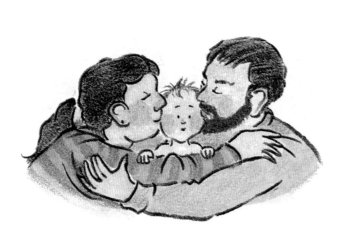

18
Instructions from Mum and Dad
The Cell: Genes and Chromosomes

All living creatures start out as a single cell. When two sex cells – an egg and a sperm – unite into a single cell, they carry all the information required to make a new baby – a new human being. This information is stored in more than one hundred thousand genes in the centre of the cell.

Some scientists describe genes as little packages of instructions. Your genes helped to decide all sorts of things about you – whether you are female or male, the colour of your eyes, the shape of your ears, the type and colour of your hair, and the colour of your skin.

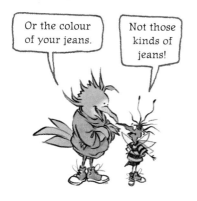

Or the colour of your jeans.

Not those kinds of jeans!

Your genes were passed on to you from both your parents, and through them from their parents, and through them from earlier generations on both sides

of your family. And many of your genes will be passed on to your children and grandchildren. If you were adopted, your genes were passed on to you by the woman and man – called your "birth mother" and your "birth father" or your "birth parents"– whose egg and sperm joined together to make you.

Genes are made of DNA – a short name for a chemical called deoxyribonucleic acid. Genes are carried on long, thread-like strings of DNA called chromosomes. A gene is a tiny part of a chromosome. A chromosome is the part of each cell that carries a person's genes. You might picture a chromosome as a string of beads, with each bead as a gene.

A chromosome

Cells in the human body usually have forty-six chromosomes. But each egg cell and each sperm cell carries only twenty-three chromosomes. If an egg and a sperm unite, the combined single cell has a grand total of forty-six chromosomes.

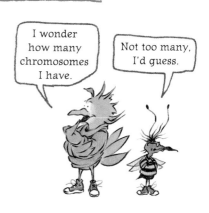

I wonder how many chromosomes I have.

Not too many, I'd guess.

That means half your chromosomes, as well as half your DNA, come from your mother and the other half come from your father. You received a combination of genes from both of them. While you are not an exact copy of either one of your parents, you probably do resemble each of them in some ways, but not in all ways.

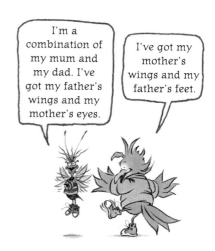

I'm a combination of my mum and my dad. I've got my father's wings and my mother's eyes.

I've got my mother's wings and my father's feet.

If two eggs leave the ovaries at the same time, and if each egg is fertilized by a separate sperm, fraternal, or non-identical, twins begin. Since fraternal twins do not have the same genes, they do not look exactly like each other and can be the same sex or the opposite sex.

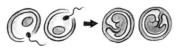

2 eggs + 2 sperm   Fraternal twins

Identical twins begin if a single egg splits into two after it has been fertilized. Since identical twins have the same genes, they are always the same sex and look almost exactly like each other.

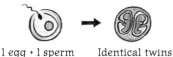

1 egg + 1 sperm   Identical twins

When two or more babies are born at the same birth – twins, triplets, and so on – it is called a multiple birth.

Unless you are an identical twin, you are not an exact genetic copy of your brother or sister, because a different sperm and egg unite to form every new baby. Each sperm and each egg carries a different combination of genes. That's why you can look a little bit different or very different from your sister or brother.

Scientists have discovered that a person's gender – female or male – is determined the moment the egg and sperm unite.

Among the twenty-three chromosomes in each egg cell and each sperm cell is one sex chromosome. There are two kinds of sex chromosomes – either an X or a Y. All eggs carry an X chromosome and all sperm carry either an X or a Y chromosome.

If an egg is fertilized by a sperm with a Y chromosome, the united single cell will develop into a baby boy – XY. And if an egg is fertilized by a sperm with an X chromosome, the united single cell will develop into a baby girl – XX.

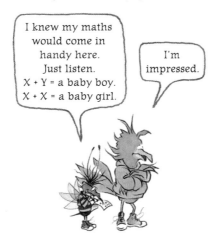

I knew my maths would come in handy here. Just listen. X + Y = a baby boy. X + X = a baby girl.

I'm impressed.

Whether you are male or female was determined by which chromosome – an X or a Y – was in the sperm from your father that fertilized your mother's egg.

The genes inside your body carry lots of information about you and determine many things – but not everything – about you.

I'm one of a kind.

Thank goodness for that.

Where you are brought up and how you are brought up, including the kind of food you eat and the kind of exercise you get, as well as the people who are around you and the events that occur as you grow up, also help to shape many things about you. That's why no two people in the world – even identical twins – are exactly alike. Each of us is unique.

19
A Kind of Sharing
Cuddling, Kissing, Touching and Sexual Intercourse

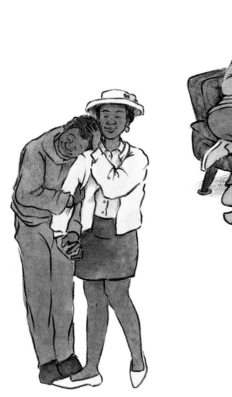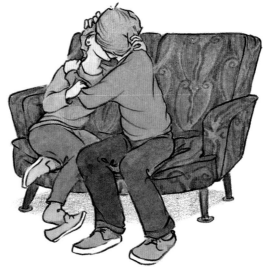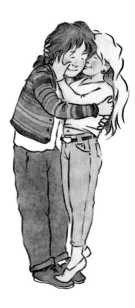

Sexual intercourse, or as it is often called, "making love", is a kind of sharing between two people. The very beginnings of a new human being – a baby – can form, immediately after sexual intercourse, if a sperm cell joins with an egg cell.

Touching, caressing, kissing, and hugging – often called "petting" – are other kinds of sharing that can make two people feel very close and loving and excited about one another. People can and do become sexually excited without having sexual intercourse. Choosing to wait to have sexual intercourse until one is older or feels more responsible is called "post-ponement". Choosing not to have sexual intercourse is called "abstinence".

When two people feel they are too young to have sexual intercourse, do not know each other well enough, or do not want to have sexual intercourse for any other reason, they may decide just to hold hands, cuddle, dance or kiss.

Sharing between two people who care about each other always means having respect for each other's feelings and wishes. This includes respecting each other's right to say "No!" to any kind of sexual activity – at any time and for any reason.

Sexual intercourse usually begins with two people touching, caressing, kissing and hugging each other.

After a bit, the female's vagina becomes moist and slippery, her clitoris becomes hard, and the male's penis becomes erect, stiff, and larger. Sometimes a bit of clear fluid that may contain a few sperm comes out of the tip of the penis and makes it wet. And the two people begin to feel excited about each other.

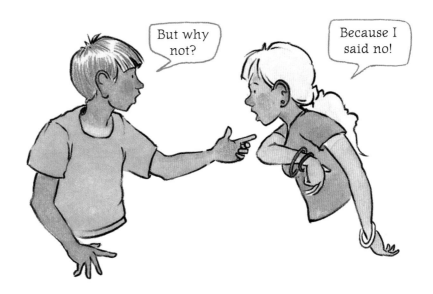

But why not?

Because I said no!

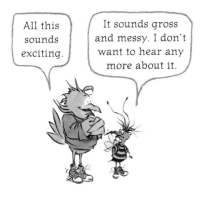

All this sounds exciting.

It sounds gross and messy. I don't want to hear any more about it.

When the two people are a male and a female, it is now possible for the male's erect penis to go inside the female's vagina, which stretches in a way that fits around the penis. The moisture from the vagina makes it easier for the penis to go in.

This kind of sexual intercourse is called "vaginal intercourse". It is also called "vaginal sex". As the male and female move back and forth in rhythm, the movement of the penis inside the vagina soon feels very good. The female and male may hug and kiss and touch each other even more as all of this is going on and feel more and more excited.

When these feelings come to a climax, semen is ejaculated from the penis and spurts into the vagina, and the muscles in the vagina and uterus tighten and finally relax. A small amount of fluid may come out of the vagina. This is called "having an orgasm".

A female and male may have orgasms at different times. And sometimes one person has an orgasm and the other doesn't. After an orgasm, most people feel relaxed, content and sometimes even sleepy.

Every time a couple has vaginal intercourse it can result in a baby – unless the female is already pregnant.

People have a lot of mistaken ideas about how a girl or woman who has had vaginal intercourse can and cannot become pregnant. It's important to know that a girl or woman can become pregnant even if she is standing up during vaginal intercourse; even if it is the very first time she has had vaginal intercourse; even if she has had vaginal intercourse only once; even if she thinks or feels she is

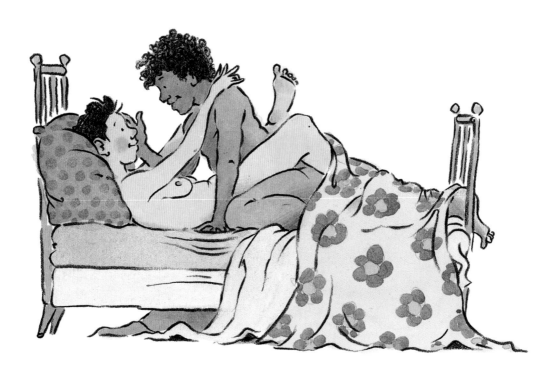

menstruating; even if she does not have an orgasm.

A girl or woman can also become pregnant even if the boy or man pulls out before he ejaculates. If sperm are ejaculated close to the opening of the vagina – or even if just a few sperm spurt out before ejaculation – it is possible for them to swim up the vagina and join with an egg. This can also happen even when a female and a male do not have vaginal intercourse, if sperm are ejaculated close to the opening of the vagina.

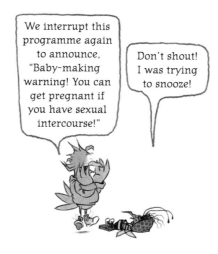

We interrupt this programme again to announce, "Baby-making warning! You can get pregnant if you have sexual intercourse!"

Don't shout! I was trying to snooze!

Waiting to have sex until one is old enough to take good care of a baby makes good sense. The surest way not to become pregnant is to abstain from – not have – vaginal sex.

However, if a female and a male decide to have sexual intercourse, there are ways – called contraception – that can help protect them from becoming pregnant and having a baby. And a couple can help protect each other from getting infections such as HIV, HPV, and gonorrhoea that are spread by sexual contact if they use a new condom correctly and every time they have sex. This is one way of practising "safer sex".

There are other ways people

make love and have sex. When a person puts his or her mouth on a female's vulva or on a male's penis, this is called "oral sex" or "oral intercourse". When a male's penis goes inside another person's anus, this is called "anal sex" or "anal intercourse".

Some think that when people have oral sex or anal sex, they are not having sex – and that they are abstaining from sex. But having oral or anal sex are not ways of abstaining from sex. They are ways of "having sex".

A female cannot become pregnant after having oral or anal sex. But anyone – female or male – can get infections such as HIV, HPV and gonorrhoea, all of which are spread by sexual contact, by having vaginal or oral or anal sex. Using a new condom or barrier correctly and every time a person has vaginal or oral or anal sex is a way of practising "safer sex".

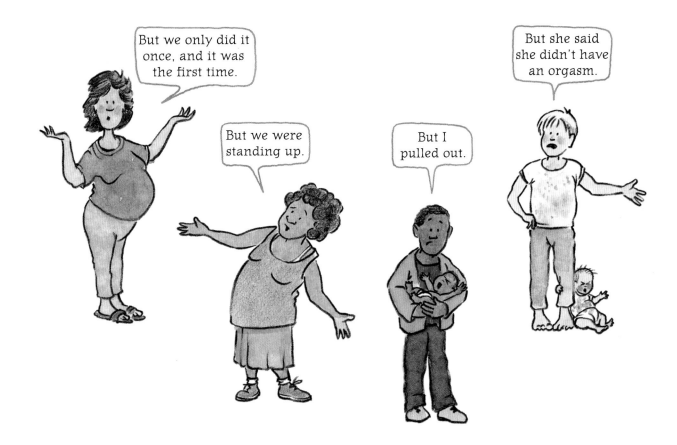

20
Before Birth
Pregnancy

The word *pregnant* comes from two Latin words: *prae*, which means *before*, and *gnas*, which means *birth.*

Pregnancy is the period of time before birth during which a fertilized egg plants itself inside the lining of the uterus, grows inside the uterus, and eventually develops into a baby. The union of a sperm and an egg is called conception or fertilization.

Scientists have discovered exactly how a pregnancy begins by observing how sperm travel, meet, and unite with an egg.

Living sperm are great travellers, and it is wonderful to watch them move under a microscope. You can actually see their tails move rapidly back and forth. They look like tadpoles swimming and travel like a school of fish – in large groups of about five hundred million.

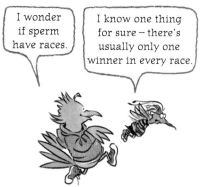

I wonder if sperm have races.

I know one thing for sure – there's usually only one winner in every race.

When sperm are ejaculated in the female's vagina during sexual intercourse, they swim up the vagina, through the cervix, into the uterus and into the Fallopian tubes. If an egg has been released and swept into one of the Fallopian tubes, a sperm can unite with it and fertilize it – and the female can become pregnant.

Only about two hundred sperm out of the five hundred million in an ejaculation get close to the egg.

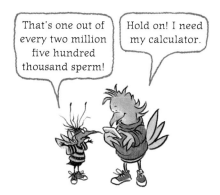

That's one out of every two million five hundred thousand sperm!

Hold on! I need my calculator.

Scientists have shown that a chemical in the fluid around the egg actually attracts certain sperm, telling them that the egg is ready, and lets only one sperm out of those two hundred or so break into the egg cell.

After that sperm enters the egg, none of the others can get in, and fertilization takes place.

Once an egg cell unites with a sperm cell, it becomes a single cell – the first cell of a baby. A fertilized egg cell is called a zygote from conception and for the next several days as it travels to the uterus; an embryo during the next two months as it develops in the uterus; and a fetus throughout the rest of the pregnancy – until a baby is born. Some people call the fetus a "developing baby".

The fertilized egg cell takes about five days to travel through the Fallopian tube and into the uterus, dividing again and again. Inside the uterus, it plants itself in the uterus's lining, where it will grow and develop into a baby. The uterus is also called "the womb".

While in the uterus, a fertilized egg cell continues to divide billions and billions of times to make billions and billions of new cells. Eventually, over nine months, these cells become a whole new person – a baby.

THE FURTHER ADVENTURES OF THE EGG AND SPERM: *Pregnancy*

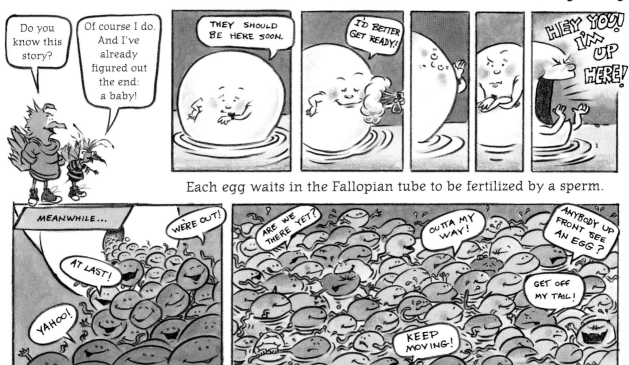

Each egg waits in the Fallopian tube to be fertilized by a sperm.

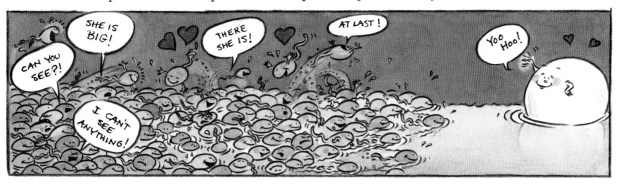

Sperm leave the penis, swim up the vagina, through the uterus,

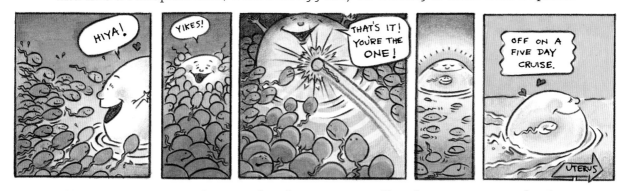

and into a Fallopian tube, where an egg may be waiting to unite with a sperm.

If one sperm enters the egg, they become one cell and pregnancy can begin.

From Zygote to Baby – 9 Months

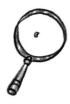
Zygote – *day 1*

Embryo – *month 1*

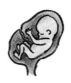
Fetus – *month 3*

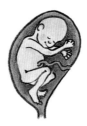
Fetus – *month 6*

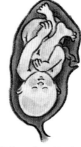
Baby about to be born – *month 9*

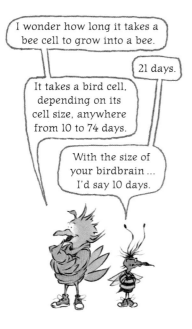

> I wonder how long it takes a bee cell to grow into a bee.

> 21 days.

> It takes a bird cell, depending on its cell size, anywhere from 10 to 74 days.

> With the size of your birdbrain ... I'd say 10 days.

A lot of children and even some grown-ups think that the developing baby grows in the mother's stomach. It does not grow in the stomach.

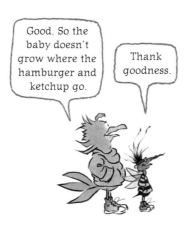

> Good. So the baby doesn't grow where the hamburger and ketchup go.

> Thank goodness.

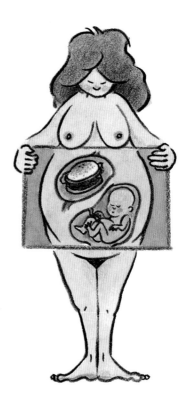

In the uterus, a sac filled with a watery fluid forms around the developing baby and protects it against pokes, bumps, and jolts. The sac is called the amniotic sac or the "waters", and the fluid is called amniotic fluid. This fluid is warm and keeps the developing baby warm as it floats.

It grows in the uterus. As the developing baby grows bigger, the uterus also grows bigger.

As the embryo fastens itself to the inside of the uterus, a special organ called the placenta forms inside the uterus. During pregnancy, the placenta supplies the embryo and – later on – the fetus with oxygen from the air the mother breathes and nutrients from the food she eats.

Nutrients are made up of vitamins, proteins, fats, sugars, carbohydrates and water – all the things a fetus needs in order to grow into a healthy baby.

The umbilical cord – a soft, bendable tube – connects the placenta to the fetus at the umbilicus. The word *umbilicus* means navel, and *navel* is another word for "tummy button".

Oxygen and nutrients travel from the placenta to the fetus in the blood that flows through the umbilical cord. The oxygen and nutrients, as well as other substances from the mother, pass from her blood into the fetus's blood.

The fetus's waste – liquids and solids that are left over from the nutrients not used by the fetus – travels back through the umbilical cord to the placenta and passes into the mother's blood. The fetus's waste leaves the mother's body along with the mother's waste.

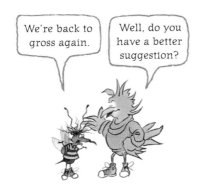

We're back to gross again.

Well, do you have a better suggestion?

Medicines, drugs, and alcohol can also pass into the fetus's blood from the mother's blood. That's why a pregnant female should be very careful about what she eats, drinks and puts into her body. If she needs to take a prescription drug, she should check with her doctor or nurse to make sure the drug will not hurt the fetus.

If a female has abused drugs, consumed alcohol, smoked cigarettes, not eaten healthy foods, or had certain kinds of infections while pregnant, her baby could be born with or develop serious health problems. It could have difficulty eating and breathing and growing properly. And if a pregnant mother has been addicted to drugs, her baby may be born addicted to drugs.

However, if a pregnant mother takes good care of herself – has regular check-ups with a nurse or doctor, eats healthy food, and gets enough exercise and sleep – her baby will have the best chance of being born healthy.

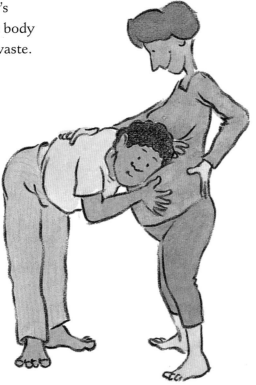

21
What a Trip!
Birth

The birth of a baby is almost always a healthy and joyful event. A pregnant woman knows that her baby is ready to be born when she can feel the muscles of her uterus tighten and squeeze and then relax, over and over, many times in a row.

The woman's muscles are actually beginning to push the baby out of her uterus. All this tightening and squeezing and pushing is called labour. *Labour* is another word for *work*.

When labour starts, the pregnant woman usually goes to a hospital unless she has arranged to have the birth at home with a doctor or a midwife and a nurse. A midwife – a person who has been specially trained to help a woman deliver a baby – is not a doctor but may be a nurse. Fathers, and sometimes other family members and friends, can also help the mother during labour and birth. Labour can be as short as an hour or longer than a whole day.

After labour has started, and occasionally before, the amniotic sac – the bag of waters – breaks, and fluid begins to leak out.

This can be another sign that the baby is ready to be born.

During the birth, the baby travels out of the uterus, through the cervix, which has opened and widened during labour, and into the vagina. The vagina stretches as the baby travels through it and out of the mother's body. The vagina is often called the "birth canal", because *canal* is another word for *passageway*.

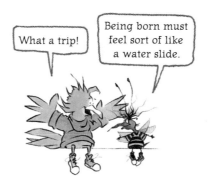

In most births, the baby's head pushes out of the vagina first. Any fluid in its mouth or nose is carefully taken out so the baby can breathe on its own. Then the rest of its body comes out. Usually the doctor, midwife, or father gently holds the newborn baby as it comes out. This is called a vaginal birth.

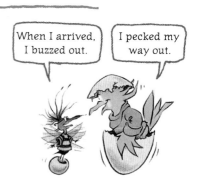

Some babies need to be gently pulled out by tongs, called forceps. This is called a forceps birth. And some babies come out of the uterus and vagina feet first. This is called a breech birth.

Other babies are too big to travel safely through the vagina. Or they are in positions that make it difficult for them to travel out of the uterus and through the vagina on their own.

If the baby is too big or in an awkward position, the doctor makes a side-to-side cut through the mother's skin – after it has been made numb with a special medicine – into the mother's uterus and lifts the baby out and cuts the umbilical cord. Then the doctor takes the placenta out and sews up the mother's cut, which heals in a few weeks' time.

WHAT A TRIP!: *Birth*

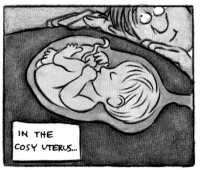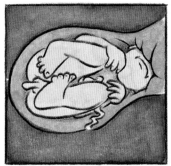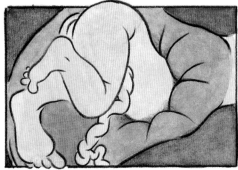

When it's time to be born, the mother's muscles squeeze and push the baby out

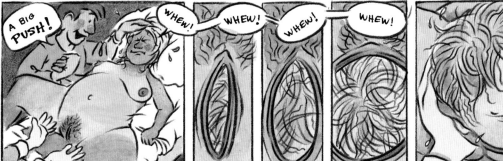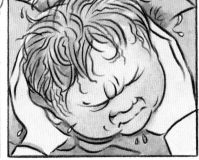

and into the vagina. The vagina stretches wide and out comes

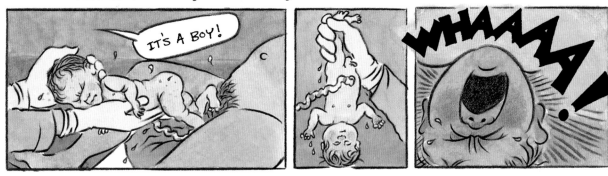

the baby, who is still connected to the mother by the umbilical cord,

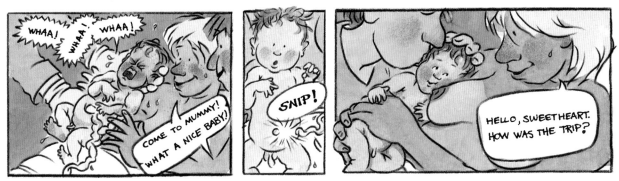

which is cut. And right away, the new baby is cuddled and held.

This is called a Caesarean birth, or "c-section", and is another healthy way for a baby to be born. It is believed that the term *Caesarean* dates back to the time of Julius Caesar, the great Roman leader, general, and politician, who may have been born this way around 100 B.C. – more than two thousand years ago.

A forceps birth, a breech birth, and a Caesarean birth are perfectly normal ways for a baby to be born. No matter which way a baby is born, right after birth it takes its first breath and lets out its first cry. This allows its lungs to open up and begin to work on their own. The moment of birth is so exciting!

Even though the baby is still attached to the placenta by the umbilical cord, it does not need the placenta anymore.

The doctor or midwife places a clamp on the baby's umbilical cord and then cuts the cord about an inch from the baby's navel. Since there are no nerve endings in the umbilical cord, neither the baby nor the mother can feel the cut.

A few days later, the clamped piece of umbilical cord dries out and falls off painlessly. The place where it was attached becomes a person's navel, or tummy button.

After the cord has been cut, the muscles of the uterus give a few more squeezes and pushes, and the placenta and amniotic sac slide out. Because they leave the mother's body after the baby has been born, they are called the afterbirth.

As soon as possible, the newborn baby is gently dried off, wrapped in a blanket, and given to the mother or father to cuddle and hold.

When parents are first given their newborn baby to hold and can feel the baby's skin against their skin and can feel the baby breathe, they have – more often than not – new and special feelings of love and awe. These fond and loving feelings between parents and their child often begin at birth, but they can also begin in the weeks after birth.

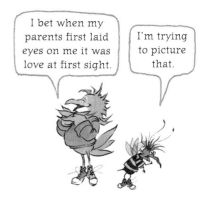

I bet when my parents first laid eyes on me it was love at first sight.

I'm trying to picture that.

A newborn baby is usually weighed and measured and given some eye drops to prevent infection a few minutes after it is born.

The birth of a baby is a fascinating event. At birth, a baby can see, hear, cry, suck, grab, feel and smell. And it can eat by sucking from its mother's breast or from a bottle. A newborn baby can do an amazing number of things.

If a boy baby is to be circumcised, that is, if the foreskin of his penis is to be removed, either by a doctor

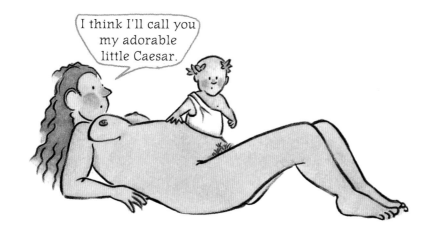

I think I'll call you my adorable little Caesar.

or a person who learned to perform circumcision as part of a religious ceremony, it is usually done a few days after birth. It takes only a few minutes to perform a circumcision.

Some circumcisions are performed for religious reasons. Baby boys who are born into the Jewish or Muslim faith are usually circumcised as part of a religious ceremony.

Other circumcisions are performed for health reasons – to make it easier to keep the tip of the penis clean by washing it with soap and water so as to prevent infections. A baby boy's or a young boy's uncircumcised penis can also be kept clean by simply washing the penis with soap and water.

When boys who have an uncircumcised penis grow older, the foreskin separates from the tip of the penis. Once that happens, an older boy's uncircumcised penis can be kept clean by gently pulling back the foreskin and washing the tip with soap and water while taking a bath or shower.

Some parents like the idea of having their son look like his father, and sometimes that's how they make the decision about whether their baby boy is going to be circumcised.

Babies are born in many different ways. Some babies are born early, before they have spent a full nine months in the uterus. This is called a premature birth. A baby who is born early is called a premature baby or a "prem baby".

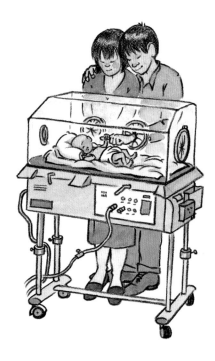

A baby who is born only two or three weeks early has grown big enough to have a healthy start in life and can usually go home with its parents after one or two days in the hospital. But if a baby is born a month or more early, living outside the uterus can be hard. The baby's lungs may not be fully developed, making it difficult for the baby to breathe. The baby may not be able to suck or swallow easily, making it difficult for the baby to eat. And the baby may have trouble staying warm.

A baby who is born a month or more early usually has to stay in the hospital until he or she is healthy enough to go home. In the hospital, the baby stays in a specially equipped cot called an incubator, which keeps the baby warm and provides oxygen – just as the mother's uterus did for the fetus – while it continues to grow. While the baby is in the incubator, the baby's parents, the doctors, and the nurses feed and take care of the baby.

When the baby has grown big enough and is close to being as healthy as a baby who has spent a full nine months growing in the uterus, and can eat well and keep warm, its parents can take their baby home.

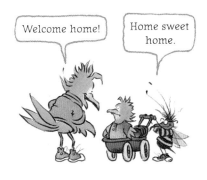

Welcome home!

Home sweet home.

22

Other Arrivals
More Ways to Have a Baby and Family

Sometimes people want to have a baby but cannot have one because their egg and sperm are not able to unite. Fortunately, there are ways other than sexual intercourse to have a baby.

There can be many different reasons why an egg cell and a sperm cell are not able to unite, such as a female's ovaries not releasing an egg each month, an egg being unable to travel through the Fallopian tubes, too few sperm travelling to the egg, or the sperm being too weak to travel to the egg.

However, with the help of a doctor, a female's egg can be fertilized by a male's sperm and a pregnancy can begin.

An egg can be taken out of one of the ovaries by a doctor and put into a small glass dish filled with fluid along with sperm that have been ejaculated. After the egg has been fertilized by one of the sperm in the dish, the egg is returned to the uterus, and a pregnancy can begin. This method of starting a pregnancy is called *in vitro* fertilization. *In vitro* are the Latin words for *in a glass*.

When a female's eggs cannot be fertilized, she may choose to have an egg from another female's ovaries put into a dish with sperm so that the egg can be fertilized. The fertilized egg is then put into the first female's uterus so that a pregnancy can begin. This is called egg donation.

When there are not enough sperm, or not enough sperm strong enough to swim to the egg, a doctor can place the male's ejaculated sperm in the female's vagina or uterus with a syringe. In the uterus, the sperm have a shorter distance to swim and a better chance of uniting with an egg in one of the Fallopian tubes.

Starting a pregnancy this way, by placing sperm from a male into a female's vagina or uterus, is called artificial insemination – even though there is nothing artificial about the egg and sperm or the uniting of the egg and sperm. *Inseminate* means *to put a seed in*, and in this case, *to make pregnant*. This is also called alternative insemination because it is an alternative

way – another way – to become pregnant.

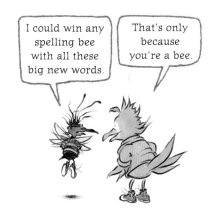

I could win any spelling bee with all these big new words.

That's only because you're a bee.

Sometimes, if a male becomes very ill, the medication he needs to become well may decrease the number of sperm that he is able to make. Before the male takes the medication, his ejaculated sperm can be placed in a sperm bank – a medical laboratory – to be frozen and stored for up to ten or fifteen years. They can be used later to conceive a baby by artificial insemination. Some healthy men also donate their sperm to a sperm bank to be used at a later date to help start a pregnancy.

Sometimes, if a female becomes very ill, she may have

her eggs removed by a doctor before she takes medication. Her eggs are then frozen and stored, and if she chooses, used later to conceive a baby by in vitro fertilization. A healthy female who wants to wait until she is older to have a baby may also have her eggs frozen to be used, if she chooses, at a later date to conceive a baby by in vitro fertilization.

Some women who are not able to conceive a baby may choose to have a surrogate pregnancy. One kind of surrogate pregnancy happens when a woman has an egg removed from her uterus by a doctor, and placed with a sperm from a male, who may or may not be her husband or partner, in a small dish in a medical laboratory – where the egg and the sperm can meet and grow into an embryo. That embryo is then implanted in another woman's uterus, where it grows into a baby. This woman is called a surrogate. Another kind of surrogate pregnancy happens when the egg that joins with the donated sperm is the surrogate's egg.

Legal documents are made and signed before either of these processes start, so that when that baby is born, the baby goes home with and is the child of the woman and man whose egg, or whose surrogate's egg, and sperm first joined together to make that baby. Or the baby is the child of and goes home with the two women, or the two men, or the single woman, or the single man who has chosen to have a surrogate pregnancy as their way to have a baby.

There are people who are not able to conceive a baby at all – by sexual intercourse, by in vitro fertilization, or by artificial insemination. Or they do not choose to have a surrogate pregnancy. But they can start a family by adopting a baby or child.

Adoption means that a family will bring another family's baby or child into their family and raise that child as their very own.

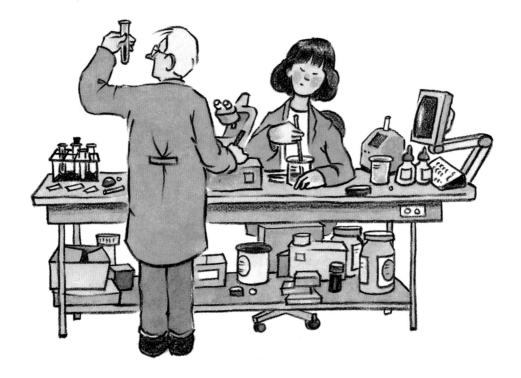

An adopted child becomes a member of his or her new family.

Many people choose to adopt children because they are not able to conceive a baby. Some people who can conceive a baby also choose to adopt children.

Adoption usually occurs when a parent or parents who are unable to take care of their newborn baby or child decide to have someone else care for, bring up, and love their baby or child.

Adoption is a legal act. This means that the child's birth parent or parents sign a paper in front of a lawyer or judge that says that they are giving their child for ever to a parent or parents who want to and are able to take care of the child. The new adoptive parent or parents agree to raise the child as their own. They too sign the adoption paper in front of a lawyer or judge.

There are many ways to have a baby and create a family. But no matter how people have a child, caring for and loving one can be a wonderful and amazing experience.

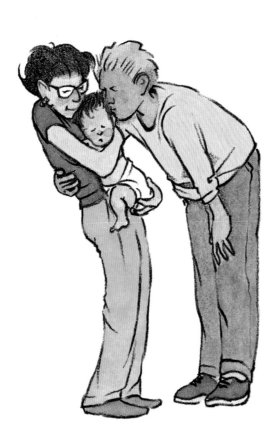

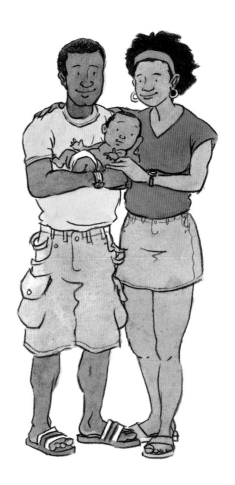

PART FIVE

Decisions

23

Planning Ahead
Postponement, Abstinence and Contraception

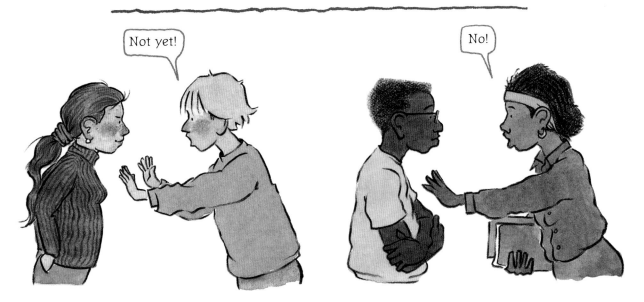

Whether or not to have sexual intercourse is a decision each person has a right to make. But a person should always remember that vaginal intercourse can result in pregnancy and having a baby. A person should also remember that vaginal, oral or anal intercourse can result in a person becoming infected with a disease, even very serious diseases.

Many young people choose to wait to have sexual intercourse until they feel they are either old enough or responsible enough to make healthy decisions about sex. This is called "postponement". *Postponement* means *to delay until a later time*. But the only sure way not to have an unwanted pregnancy is to not have vaginal intercourse. The only sure way not to get infected is to not have sexual contact with another person. Not having sex is called "abstinence". *Abstinence* means *to abstain, to keep from doing something you want to do.*

Postponement and abstinence can prevent the start of a pregnancy and can also help prevent a person from getting or passing on infections that are spread by sexual contact. These kinds of infections are called sexually transmitted diseases or sexually transmitted infections. They are also called STDs or STIs for short.

Many people who choose to postpone or abstain from

sexual intercourse say that they can still have a close, loving and sexy relationship with another person.

Sometimes, when people choose to have vaginal intercourse, they have planned to have a baby. But other people may want to wait to have a baby or may not want to have a baby at all. That's why knowing how to prevent pregnancy is important.

Family planning, birth control and *contraception* are the names given to the many ways of preventing a pregnancy.

Contra is the Latin word for *against. Ception* is part of the word *conception*, which means *beginning. Contraception* means *against beginning a pregnancy.*

There are many kinds of contraception, and some work better than others. For most kinds, a person must learn how to use them correctly and every time he or she has sexual intercourse in order for them to work. However, no method of contraception can be guaranteed to work 100 percent of the time.

If a person makes the decision to have sexual intercourse, the most useful protection against pregnancy is the correct use of contraception before or at the time of sexual intercourse. It's important to know and

remember that using any type of contraception can help to prevent a pregnancy and most often it does prevent a pregnancy. But using ANY type of contraception without ALSO using a condom does not protect a couple from getting or passing on a sexually transmitted disease. That's why a couple must also use a condom. It's also important to know and remember that the best protection from becoming infected with a sexually transmitted disease AND from becoming pregnant is for a couple to use a condom WITH another type of contraception.

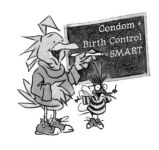

Most contraceptive methods are free from sexual health clinics and some family doctors. You can talk to a doctor or a health professional about any method and your talk will be confidential. Condoms are sold widely (in pharmacies, supermarkets, some garages and online).

A male condom is a soft, very thin cover that fits over an erect

penis. When a male ejaculates, semen is kept inside the condom and sperm are not able to enter the vagina and unite with an egg.

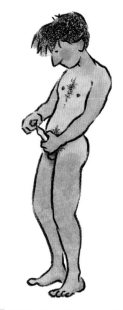

Putting on a male condom

Condoms are also called "johnnies" or "rubbers" because they are usually made out of a rubbery material called latex. There are other types of male condoms made out of rubbery materials called polyurethane and polyisoprene. It is important to use a latex, polyurethane, or polyisoprene condom – not a lambskin condom. Viruses that are transmitted by sexual contact, such as HIV and hepatitis B can seep through the tiny pores in the lambskin and cause a person to become infected.

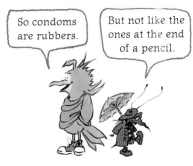

So condoms are rubbers.

But not like the ones at the end of a pencil.

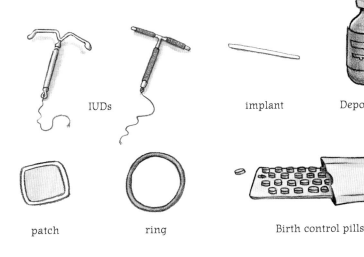

IUDs

implant

Depo-Provera

patch

ring

Birth control pills

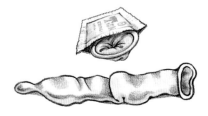

Male condom

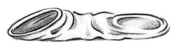

Female condom

A condom designed to fit inside the vagina, called the female condom, is often made out of polyurethane. This soft pouchlike condom is inserted into the vagina before sexual intercourse.

Using a new condom during sexual intercourse, correctly and every time, can also help prevent the spread of infections – mild infections as well as more serious infections such as HIV and hepatitis B. This is a way of practicing safer sex. The most common infection that can be passed on is chlamydia. Although chlamydia is not life-threatening, it can cause infertility so that a female will not be able to become pregnant in the future and have a baby. It's important to understand that any type of birth control method, when used by itself – *without* a condom – *cannot* prevent a person from getting an infection from or passing on an infection to another person.

It is also important to use condoms with silicone- or water-based lubricants made especially for sex, and *not* made with oil. Oil can damage and break a latex condom.

The IUD, IUS, the implant, and the contraceptive injection are the most effective kinds of contraception. The pill, the patch, and the ring are almost as effective. Other kinds of birth control can also be effective, but are not quite as effective.

The IUD, IUS, the contraceptive injection, the implant, contraceptive pills, the patch, the ring, the cervical cap, and the diaphragm are all contraceptives that a female can obtain only after visiting her family doctor or a sexual health clinic and obtaining a written prescription. The prescribed contraceptive method can then be obtained at a chemist or health clinic.

IUDs (intra-uterine devices) and IUSs (intra-uterine systems) are small devices that are placed inside the uterus by a trained health-care professional and affect the way sperm move – so that sperm cannot swim to and join with an egg.

The implant and contraceptive injection are contraceptive methods that contain artificial hormones that keep the ovaries from releasing eggs. The implant, a thin, flexible plastic-like rod, about the

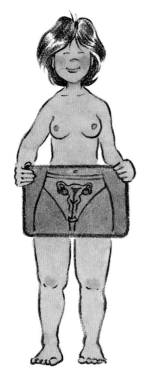

size of a cardboard matchstick, can be inserted by a health professional under the skin of a female's upper arm and can stay in for three years. It can also make the fluid around the cervix thicker – keeping a sperm from joining an egg. The contraceptive injection is injected in a female's upper arm or buttocks every three months.

Contraceptive pills, commonly called "the pill", contain artificial hormones that keep ovaries from releasing eggs. A female must remember to follow the directions for taking a pill each day for this method to work.

The patch and the ring contain and release artificial hormones that can keep the ovaries from releasing eggs. The patch is a thin, square patch of plastic that sticks to the skin and looks like a bandage. It is placed by a female on the skin of her upper arm, upper torso, stomach, or buttocks – but should not be placed on the breasts. Each week for three weeks, a new patch is placed on the female's body. The fourth week, no patch is used. The next month, the same process begins again. The ring is a

Where They Fit

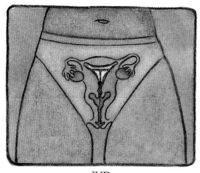

IUD

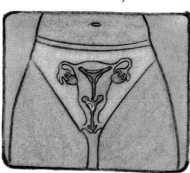

Ring

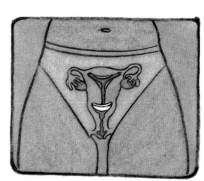

Diaphragm

Cervical cap

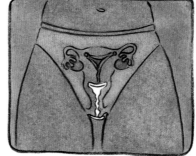

Female condom

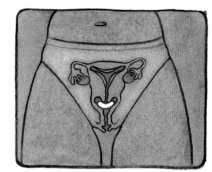

Sponge

small, soft, flexible plastic ring a female inserts into her vagina. It is left in place for three weeks, and then is removed for one week. After that week, the female inserts a new ring.

The cervical cap and diaphragm are small rubbery cups that fit inside the vagina and are placed against the cervix before sexual intercourse. Both can prevent sperm from entering the cervix and travelling to the Fallopian tubes. And both must be used with a spermicide.

Spermicide comes in different forms – foams, creams, jellies and gels. The chemical in spermicide can kill sperm. Sponges containing spermicide may also block sperm and keep them from joining an egg. These kinds of contraceptives are inserted into the vagina before sexual intercourse. But they are not always able to kill, block or catch every sperm and do not

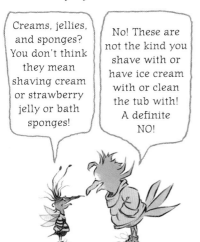

Creams, jellies, and sponges? You don't think they mean shaving cream or strawberry jelly or bath sponges!

No! These are not the kind you shave with or have ice cream with or clean the tub with! A definite NO!

protect a person from getting or passing on an infection.

Spermicide should *not* be used if a person is having intercourse often or having anal sex. Either may cause irritation that could increase the risk of infection. Spermicide and sponges can be bought at a chemist or supermarket. They are often displayed in a special section, and no prescription is needed. They can also be bought online.

If there is an emergency and a woman or girl has been raped – forced to have sex against her will – there are emergency contraceptive pills that she can take to prevent the start of a pregnancy. These pills are also called "morning-after pills". They can also be used if a condom breaks, or is not put on properly, or a patch falls off, or a woman or girl has unprotected sex for any reason. But they should not be relied upon as a regular form of birth control because there are many other kinds of methods that are more effective.

Morning-after pills contain hormones that are thought to delay ovulation and prevent the ovaries from releasing any eggs, so that pregnancy cannot begin. Some types of these pills must be taken within 72

hours – three days – after vaginal intercourse. Other types must be taken within 120 hours – five days – after vaginal intercourse. And they are more effective when taken as soon as possible after unprotected vaginal intercourse. However, any time a female has unprotected intercourse and does not want to become pregnant, she will need to take the pills again. With some brands, it is only necessary to take one pill. With other brands, it is necessary to take two pills.

Some brands of the morning-after pill can be obtained by females of any age for free from sexual health clinics, doctors, Accident & Emergency units and some special pharmacies. You have to be over sixteen to buy emergency contraception over-the-counter from other pharmacies. An IUD can also be inserted as a form of emergency contraception, and this must be done by a health-care professional.

Some methods of birth control, such as the rhythm method or the withdrawal method, are not considered effective for preventing pregnancy or STDs.

When a male and a female use the rhythm method, they try to figure out when the female's ovary has released an egg and then abstain from having vaginal intercourse during that time. However, it is very difficult to know when an egg has been released, because the time can vary from month to month – *especially* for many teenage girls.

When a couple uses the withdrawal method, the male removes his penis from the female's vagina just before he ejaculates. This method does *not* work very well either because some semen may leak out before ejaculation or because the male may fail to remove his penis before he ejaculates.

Sometimes when people decide not to have more children, they may choose to have a simple operation called sterilization.

When a male has this operation – called a vasectomy – a small piece of the vas deferens is removed or tied off by a doctor. As a result, the semen that is ejaculated no longer carries any sperm.

When a female has this operation – called a tubal ligation or a tubal sterilization – a small piece of each Fallopian tube is removed or tied off or blocked by a doctor so that an egg cannot get to the uterus and sperm cannot get to an egg.

Some religions and groups and some individuals believe that using any method of contraception is wrong. Others believe that using the rhythm method and withdrawal method is fine. However, they also believe that using over-the-counter and prescription contraception methods is wrong.

Still many others think birth control is a fine and responsible way to prevent an unwanted pregnancy or delay having a baby.

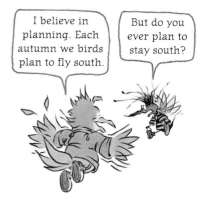

These people use contraception to help them plan a family.

Your parent or parents, a doctor or nurse are good people to talk to about contraception, postponement and abstinence. If you talk to a doctor or nurse your talk will be confidential. Sexual health clinics are also places to go for information.

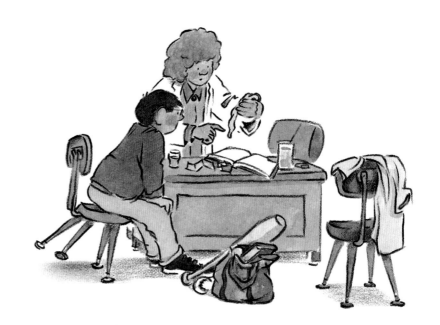

24
Laws and Rulings
Abortion

An abortion is a medical procedure performed for the purpose of ending a pregnancy. Some pregnant females choose to have abortions. People's feelings about having abortions are not always simple, however, and can range from relief to sadness, from worry to fear.

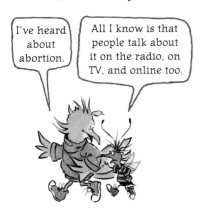

I've heard about abortion.

All I know is that people talk about it on the radio, on TV, and online too.

The word *abort* means *to stop* or *to end something at an early stage.* An abortion is performed in a clinic or a hospital by a doctor and is a safe procedure, especially when done early in the pregnancy. The pregnancy is ended by removing the embryo or fetus from the uterus. The procedure itself takes about five minutes and is usually carried out during the first three months of pregnancy, before most females even look pregnant.

There are pills that can end a pregnancy and are used as another method of abortion. They can be taken by a pregnant female during the first nine weeks of a pregnancy and require visits to a doctor's office or a clinic. The pregnant female then takes a series of pills over several days. The pills cause the lining of the uterus and the embryo to leave the female's body.

These are some, but not all, of the reasons why a female or a couple might want or need to end a pregnancy:

- The female has an illness or inherited disease that makes the pregnancy or birth dangerous to her health and might even cause her death.
- A test shows that the fetus is carrying a serious inherited disease or a serious birth defect.
- The mother or father is sick and unable to take care of a baby.
- The parents do not have enough money or time to take good care of a baby or they already have children and cannot afford another child.
- The parents feel they are too young to take care of a baby in a responsible manner.
- The female feels she was not ready to become pregnant.
- The female was forced to have sexual intercourse against her will – raped – and became pregnant as a result.
- The female is single and feels she is not able to raise a child on her own.
- The female did not intend or want to become pregnant.

People have very strong feelings about whether or not a female has the right to choose to have an abortion. In some countries, abortion is a right for all women and girls; while in others, the right to abortion is only permitted in some circumstances.

The laws about abortion vary in different parts of the UK and in different parts of the world. In the United States and Australia abortion is legal, but the circumstances under which a female can have one may vary from state to state.

In the UK there are laws which govern the circumstances under which a female can choose to have an abortion. In 1967 Parliament passed a law called The Abortion Act. This law made abortion legal in the UK and allows doctors to perform an abortion under certain circumstances:

• If continuing the pregnancy puts the female's life at risk.
• If continuing the pregnancy would damage the female's physical or emotional health.

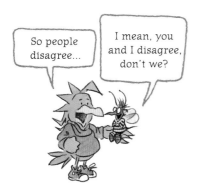

• If continuing the pregnancy would damange the physical or emotional health of a child she already has.
• If there is a considerable risk that the fetus would be born with a serious handicap.

This does not automatically give a female the right to end a pregnancy. If a female chooses to have an abortion, she must talk to two doctors. Both doctors must agree that she can have one, according to the conditions set down in The Abortion Act. Doctors may also consider her living circumstances: her housing, her income and any help she may need to bring up her baby. If both doctors agree, and the

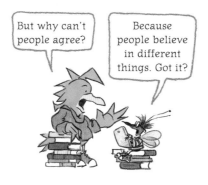

female chooses to end her pregnancy, the abortion must then be performed by a doctor in a National Health Hospital or a clinic that has been approved by the Department of Health.

The laws about a female's right to have an abortion have changed over the years and may continue to change. Scientists have discovered that a baby as early as six months can survive outside the womb. This knowledge led to a change in the 1967 Abortion Act. In 1990 the 1967 Act was revised by Parliament and a new Act – the 1990 Human Fertilisation and Embryology Act – stated that abortion can be performed at up to six months of pregnancy. Most abortions in the UK are performed before three months of a pregnancy.

If a pregnant female under the age of sixteen seeks an abortion, in most cases she must have the permission of a parent or guardian before it can be performed.

People have very strong views about the abortion laws. Those who approve of them believe a female has the right to have an abortion. Many others favour a female's right to choose for herself whether or not to have an abortion. They believe that it is a deeply personal choice that should be made by the individual female, not by the government.

People against the abortion laws believe that allowing a woman to have an abortion is wrong. They believe that life begins when a baby is con-ceived and that a fetus has a right to grow in the mother's body and to be born whether or not the mother wants to have a baby.

Because laws can and do change, and because they may vary in different places, you might want to ask your parents or teacher what the abortion laws are now, where you live.

Sometimes, usually during the early months of pregnancy, an abortion happens by itself, without a medical procedure. This is called a spontaneous abortion or a miscarriage.

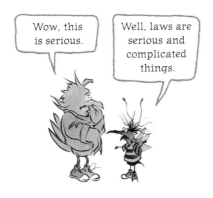

Wow, this is serious.

Well, laws are serious and complicated things.

When this happens, the embryo or fetus is released from the mother's uterus without warning, often because it is not developing normally. Doctors do not always understand why miscarriages happen, but they know that females who have miscarriages can usually become pregnant again and give birth to healthy babies. The same is true for females who have chosen to have an abortion.

PART SIX

Staying Healthy

25
Helpful – Fun – Creepy – Dangerous
Texting, Messaging, Emailing, Being Online

Many young people, but not all, have a mobile phone and keep in touch with their friends and family by texting, online chatting, calling, instant messaging (also called IM-ing), emailing, or even having a video chat. And many young people use tablets or computers to go online to contact others and to find information.

But it's important to remember that mobile phones, tablets and computers are just machines. And while these devices can provide good, fast ways to get information or to communicate with another person by texting, instant messaging, emailing, or contacting a friend online, they are not a substitute for actually being with a real person in real time. In fact, in every relationship and in every friendship, being with another person is very important.

It's also very important to know and remember that anything and everything you put in a text, or instant message, or post online is there for ever, and may not remain private if someone sends it on to or shares it with another person.

Chances are that you spend time online and that you already

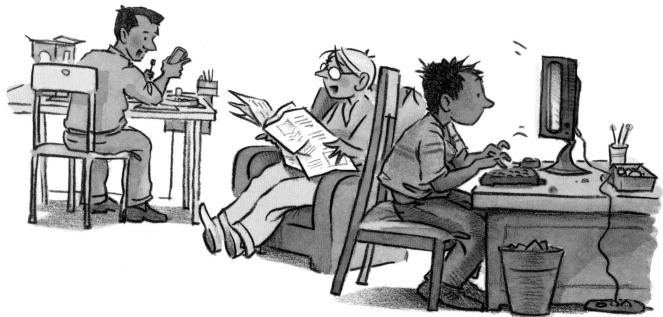

know that the Internet can be a great place to look up something you want to learn about or have questions or concerns about. You may also go online to watch videos, play games, get homework assignments, get help with homework, or to keep in touch with other people. Some of you may contact friends online by going on a social network site where friends can also communicate with one another.

Information you may find on the Internet can be very useful. Going to websites and online encyclopaedias and dictionaries can be a quick way to find information you are looking for. Searching for a word or topic online can also be helpful. Older children and teens can find lots of responsible information online – including information about bodies, puberty, sex and sexual health.

Here are some ways websites can be helpful. For example, if you are curious or have questions about puberty or HIV/AIDS, you can look up these and other topics online and learn about them. If you are the only girl in your class who has not started having periods or the only boy in your class whose voice has not changed, you can go online and most likely find out that

not getting your period yet or not having your voice change yet is perfectly normal.

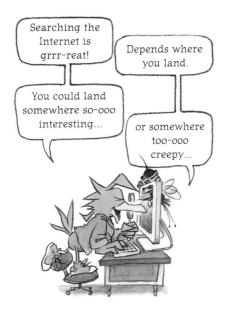

Searching the Internet is grrr-reat!

Depends where you land.

You could land somewhere so-ooo interesting...

or somewhere too-ooo creepy...

Information on the Internet about sex and bodies that is specifically written for older children and teens can also help a person make good and safe decisions about sexual health. That's because you can find facts on the Internet about topics such as the real risks of unprotected sexual contact, including pregnancy and the very real risk of being infected by a sexually transmitted disease. The Internet can also be a good place to check out if what you think you know or have heard about bodies or sex from your friends is true or not.

Here are some things you need to think about when you go on the Internet.

There can be a lot of inappropriate, weird, confusing, uncomfortable, creepy, scary or even dangerous websites that you can end up on when looking for information. This can happen if you end up on a website by accident, or on purpose, that has material you were not expecting. While some of this information can feel exciting for older children and teens, it can also feel scary, upsetting, strange, gross, troubling or puzzling. Often young people and teens have many of these feelings all at the same time, and that can also feel confusing or even disturbing.

Some websites are not always what they tell you they are. They are not real or responsible health or medical sites. And they could contain health or medical information that is scientifically or medically wrong, or information that is not up-to-date or not always true or correct.

Wrong or old information can be harmful or even dangerous. It is not safe and it may not help you to stay healthy. And it can cause you to make decisions about your body and sex that are not healthy decisions for you or your friends. That's why it's very important to check with a trusted adult – your parent, or a teacher, librarian, therapist, school counsellor, doctor, nurse, or clergyperson – to make sure the website you are going to or have just gone to has accurate and up-to-date information.

If you happen to end up on a website and you see anything or read anything that makes you feel uncomfortable in any way, remember that you have not done anything wrong. You thought you were going to a responsible website and then

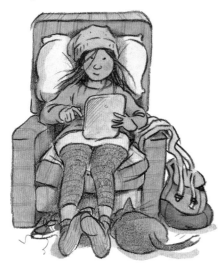

you ended up somewhere else.

You may even find yourself on a site that has photos or videos of naked bodies or sexual acts that are created to make a person feel sexually excited. Some people call these kinds of photos or videos "porn" or

"pornography". Some young people do not want to see these kinds of images at all; others are curious about them and may find them exciting. Even so, people think that young people should stay away from porn.

In some cases, passing on some kinds of porn to others can be risky and might be considered illegal. That's one reason why it's also important to talk with a trusted person if you end up on a porn site – no matter why you ended up on that site.

Whether you happen to end up on one of these sites, or on any site, by accident or on purpose – if what you see is upsetting, scary, confusing, gross and/or weird, or more than you ever want to see about bodies or sex, and makes you feel uncomfortable, leave that site right away. And talk with a person you know and trust right away. Talking with someone about what you saw and how you feel can be very helpful.

Usually, but not always, the people in these photos or videos are actors, who

are not having caring, loving, real relationships, and are not having relationships in which they treat each other with respect. What is important to know and understand is that what really matters in any relationship involving sex is that people treat one another in respectful, caring and loving ways.

No matter what, if you ever find yourself in an inappropriate or uncomfortable situation while you are on the Internet, always remember that you don't need to look at or read what is online, whether you have gone there by mistake or because you thought you wanted to be there.

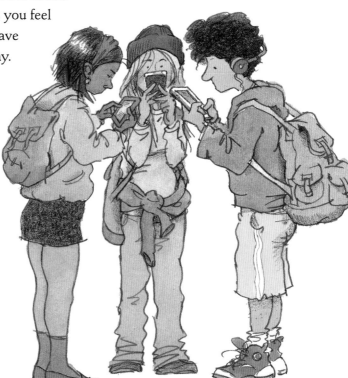

And if you read something in a text message, an instant message, or receive an email that worries you in any way, do not reply. Instead, talk with a responsible and trusted person about what you just saw or read.

Here are some rules to think about when you go online to talk to or meet someone through a social network site. Following these rules can help you protect yourself.

- Every time you use a mobile phone, a tablet, or a computer, the most important thing to think about is your privacy and safety and that of your family, friends and classmates. And whenever you set up privacy settings, it's a good idea to check in with a parent or trusted adult to help you make sure you have set up your settings in a way that protects you.

- You may think that certain sites are privacy protected, but many are not. This means that it is possible that people you know and even strangers could see posts you do not want them to see – posts you thought were private and wanted to keep private. So be sure to check the privacy settings on any site you go on.

- Only "friend" people you know. It is also extremely important to make sure that you use privacy settings to make sure that information from and about you is blocked from everyone except the people on your online "friends" list. And if someone instant messages or emails you, or says that he or she is a "buddy" or "friend" but has a screen name you do not recognize, then block that screen name so that person cannot contact you again.

- Do not post any private details about yourself, such as your age, gender, telephone number, street address, the name and street of your school, or where you are going, to anyone whom you do not know, when you visit a social network site on the Internet. If anyone asks you questions that you do not want to answer, do not answer them, and immediately tell a trusted adult. And never give anyone your password.

- If you get a call or text message on your phone and you do not know who sent it or do not recognize the telephone number, do not answer that call or text message and delete it from your phone.

- Do not have online chats with or arrange to meet someone who contacts you online whom you do not know in person, even if a friend knows that person or if the person is someone from your school whom you've never met. The same rule applies if someone you don't know instant messages or text messages you and tries to get you to come and meet them in person. Some strangers who contact you online could be grown-ups pretending to be children as a way to get you to meet them. You cannot know for sure who a stranger on the Internet really is. It's even possible that you could be physically hurt by a stranger. You need to tell a trusted adult immediately if a stranger ever contacts you online and asks to meet you in person, even if the stranger tells you to keep this a secret. Finding and telling a trusted adult can help you to stay safe.

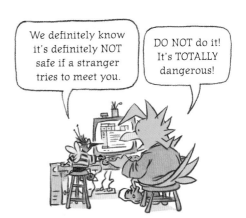

We definitely know it's definitely NOT safe if a stranger tries to meet you.

DO NOT do it! It's TOTALLY dangerous!

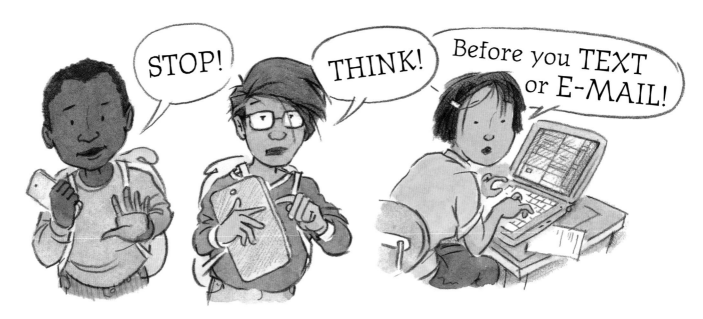

Texting or posting sexual messages, photos, or videos to someone over the Internet is called "sexting", which is a combination of two words – *sex* and *texting.* In some countries, "sexting" may be considered a crime. That is one more reason to be extremely careful about what you decide to send to someone via the Internet. It matters that you know that what you send may not remain private and what that could mean for you and your friends and family – especially something that might be considered "sexting". Thinking about this may help you to decide not to text, post, or send something that is private about you and/or your body or about any friend.

Never text, email, or post or copy videos or photos of you or your family or friends on the Internet that you would not want your parent or teacher to see. Never text, email, or post or copy a video or photo of yourself, or any part of your body, even if you think sending a picture of your belly button or a picture of you in boxer shorts or in polka-dot knickers is funny. Why not? Someone can send this video or photo to all of your classmates, even to other schools and all around the world. If just one person sends it on, it can go anywhere on the Internet, to anyone else's mobile phone, tablet, computer – to other children, to your parent, or even to your teacher or the head of your school, and even to strangers.

The same thing is true with words you may text, email, or post via the Internet. Behave as carefully online as you would in everyday contact with another person. Before you say something mean about someone or get angry with someone in a text message, post, or email, think twice before sending those strong words.

Once your words are on the Internet, they are there for ever, and you cannot get those words back. Others whom you do not want to see those words may end up seeing them. There is no way to guarantee that what you have sent will remain private.

If you say online that someone is fat or skinny or sexy or ugly or beautiful or handsome, what you have said is really never private once those words are on the Internet. Saying something mean, or bullying someone, or spreading any kind of gossip, even sexy gossip, about another person, can make that person feel really crummy and can hurt that person's feelings. When someone does this online by texting, posting, or emailing, it is called *cyber-bullying*. To *bully* means *to mistreat another person*. *Cyber-bullying* means *mistreating another person online*.

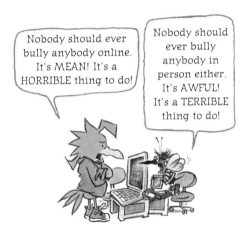

Nobody should ever bully anybody online. It's MEAN! It's a HORRIBLE thing to do!

Nobody should ever bully anybody in person either. It's AWFUL! It's a TERRIBLE thing to do!

Many parents and schools have rules about using mobile phones and the Internet. Many schools have forms to sign to make sure you follow their rules when on the Internet or on a mobile phone. These rules and forms are not about keeping you from finding information online or from being in touch with friends.

Parents and teachers have these rules and forms to keep you safe – whenever you use a mobile phone, tablet, or computer. You may wonder, safe from what? Parents, teachers and librarians are afraid that you will end up on a website that might upset or possibly harm you, and they want to stop either of those things from happening to you. These rules can help keep you safe whenever you are online or on your mobile phone. And they can help make sure that any private information about you stays private, so that strangers cannot contact you or meet you.

Every family and school may feel differently about mobile phones and the Internet and may have different rules. It's important to talk with your family about their rules and to also find out what the rules are in your school, so that you do stay safe.

Finding healthy information and staying safe on the Internet is something most everyone can do. But if you need help or come across information that's upsetting, or if someone online whom you don't know tries to meet you in person – make sure you go and talk to an adult you trust. That adult can help you to stay both healthy and safe.

Going online can be useful and interesting because of the many wonderful and responsible websites that can help you find the information you are looking for – or new or different information that you may find by chance. The information you find on responsible websites can turn out to be helpful to you by answering questions or addressing concerns you may have about sexual health. It can also help you think about yourself and your friends in new and caring ways as you are growing up and going through puberty and adolescence.

26
Talk About It
Sexual Abuse

It's sad but true that some people's sexual behaviour can be dangerous and even hurt others. This kind of behaviour is called sexual abuse.

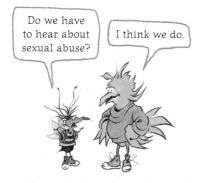

Sexual abuse is a subject that children and adults find very hard and painful to think about and talk about. People often hear a lot of wrong and confusing things about it.

Though most children have probably heard the words *sexual abuse*, that doesn't mean they know exactly what those words mean. *Sexual* means *having something to do with sex*. *Abuse* means *to treat wrongly, to mistreat*.

Sexual abuse happens when someone mistreats a person in a sexual way. Sometimes it happens when someone who is more powerful than another person or when someone who is older than another person takes advantage of that person in a sexual way. It is wrong for anyone to take advantage of another person just because he or she is older or more powerful.

Most of us – children and grown-ups – are taught rules as we are growing up about treating others with respect. Sexual abuse happens when someone breaks the rules that have to do with another person's body. When someone talks about or makes unwanted or inappropriate sexual comments to another person about that person's body – that's one kind of sexual abuse.

Sexual abuse also happens when someone touches or does something to the private parts – the sexual parts – of another person's body that that person does not want him or her to do, or when someone makes another person do something to his or her private parts that the person does not want to do.

This someone can be someone the person knows, someone the person loves, or a stranger. The truth is that it is most likely, but not always, someone the person knows. Sexual abuse can happen between children and adults – even between a parent and a child. It can also happen between one child and another child and between brothers and sisters. It can happen to both boys and girls.

The usual and normal daily hugging, kissing, touching and holding hands that go on among family members and good friends because they care about each other are not

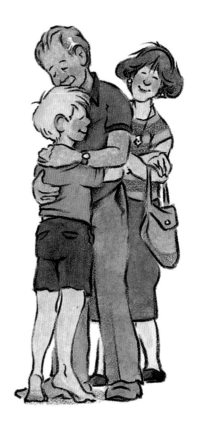

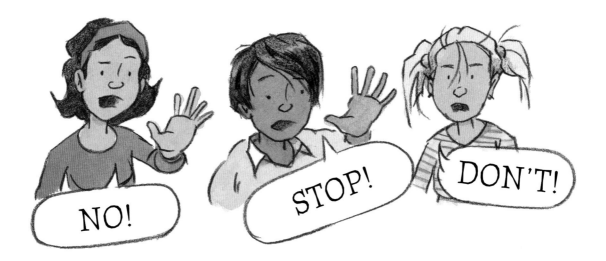

sexual abuse. A doctor's or nurse's physical examination of a person's body is not sexual abuse either. Everyone needs to have regular medical check-ups to stay healthy.

Sexual abuse can feel painful or even hurt a lot. But not all sexual abuse hurts. In fact, a person can be abused in a way that can feel loving and gentle. When this happens, a person can feel very confused, because it's almost impossible to understand how something so wrong can feel gentle or loving.

In any sexual touching or sexual relationship, every male and female – even if one person is stronger or older or more powerful than the other person – has the responsibility to have a caring, thoughtful and respectful relationship with the other person. Boys need to respect girls and girls need to respect boys by not coercing

– which means forcing – the other person to engage in any type of sexual relationship, even when one's sexual feelings are very strong.

Whether sexual abuse hurts or feels gentle or even loving, it is always wrong. People, especially grown-ups, know it is wrong. It is not your fault if it happens to you. Even if children do not know the rules, grown-ups do or should know the rules.

It is important always to remember that your body belongs to you. It's also important to know there are lots of people around who do care about children and want to keep them safe.

If anyone tries to do something to your body that you don't want them to do or don't think they should do, say, "NO!" or "STOP!" or "DON'T!" to the person who is abusing you.

Some of you may have heard

the word *harass*. Harass means *to annoy* or *bother*. If anyone harasses or bothers you by talking about sex, by using rude or dirty words about sex when you don't want them to, or by talking about your body in a way that you don't like – tell that person to STOP! Even though that person is not actually touching your body, talking about sex or your body in this way can be a kind of sexual abuse.

Sometimes a person will try to tempt another person to engage in sex by flirting or telling a person how pretty or handsome she or he is, or by dressing in a sexy manner. This can feel very confusing because there are times that these kinds of behaviours are fine and normal. But sometimes they are not fine or normal *at all* and can even include offering a person alcohol or drugs – even when that person is too young – or showing that person photos or videos of naked bodies.

These kinds of behaviours are WRONG and INAPPRO-PRIATE and they can happen to both boys and girls. If this ever happens – tell that person to STOP! And then go and tell a trusted adult as soon as you can what has happened, so that adult can help to make this stop. This too is a type of abuse.

There are some secrets with a trusted friend that are OK to keep. But don't keep sexual abuse a secret if it happens to you or to a friend – even if someone tells you to keep it a secret. Tell another person you know and trust – right away!

If the first person you tell doesn't listen to you, tell a second person. Talk about it until you find someone who understands you and believes you. That person will help you.

Always remember, if some-one abuses you, it is NEVER your fault!

You also should never abuse anyone in any way. It's not fair. It's not your right. When someone says no to you, you must believe that person and honour that person's wishes.

Most people don't like to talk about sexual abuse, but now more people are talking about it. A person can talk about it with a parent or a friend or a teacher. Very often

it helps to talk with a therapist, a school counsellor, a doctor, a nurse, or a clergy member – people specially trained to help. When a person who has been sexually abused can talk about it with someone he or she trusts, he or she may eventu-ally feel better about what has happened.

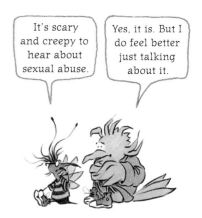

It's scary and creepy to hear about sexual abuse.

Yes, it is. But I do feel better just talking about it.

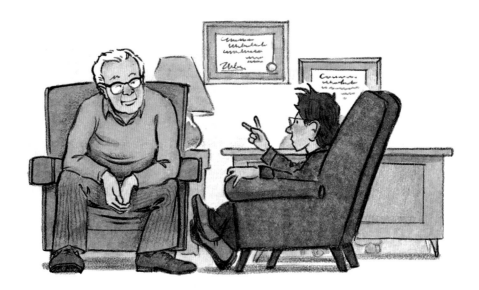

27

Getting a Check-up
Sexually Transmitted Diseases

Sex is usually a healthy, natural, and perfectly normal part of life. But sometimes sexual activities can be unhealthy.

Sexually transmitted diseases – called STDs for short – are diseases, infections, or illnesses that can spread from one person to another through sexual contact, from sexual touching to any kind of sexual intercourse – vaginal, oral, or anal intercourse. Another term for STDs is *STIs* – short for *sexually transmitted infections*. An older term for STDs is *VDs* – short for *venereal diseases*.

Infections and diseases such as colds and flus are caused by germs, which are so tiny they can be seen only by looking under a microscope. Not all germs cause illness. But some germs, including some viruses and bacteria, do. Germs can be passed from one person to another by all sorts of contact – such as sneezing, shaking hands, and using the same glass, plate or cutlery.

STDs are different from most other infections – different from colds or the flu – because they are spread by sexual contact. Most people do not like to talk about STDs.

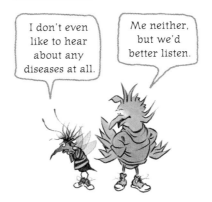

I don't even like to hear about any diseases at all.

Me neither, but we'd better listen.

There are many STDs. Some are not very serious. Others can be extremely serious; they can cause people not to be able to conceive a baby; they can even cause death. But many can be cured. And there are medicines and treatments that can make a person feel better if he or she has one of the STDs that cannot be cured.

Germs are not the only way a person can get an STD. A few STDs, such as pubic lice and scabies, are caused by tiny insects.

Pubic lice are a fairly common STD. You may have heard people call lice "crabs". That's because lice are tiny six-legged insects that look like crabs. Pubic lice like to live in warm, hairy places, like the pubic area, and are passed on through sexual contact. Pubic lice can be easily cured by putting a medicine, which kills the lice, on the pubic area. These lice are different from common head lice, because head lice are not transmitted from one person to another by sexual contact. Head lice are not an STD.

Scabies can be, but is not always, an STD. It is caused by tiny insects called mites that can cause severe itching in the areas around a person's genitals, as well as other parts of the body, except the neck and head. Scabies can be treated by putting medicine on the infected area.

Sexual contact is not the only way a person can get lice or scabies; contact with an infected person's sheets, towels or clothing can also pass them on.

Chlamydia, gonorrhoea, and syphilis are three STDs that are caused by bacteria. They can usually be cured by going to a doctor or a clinic and taking the correct medicine. However, if these STDs are not treated, a person can become very sick and lose his or her sight or the ability to have children. A mother who has one of these STDs can pass it on and cause damage to her newborn baby.

Often a person who has chlamydia or gonorrhoea does not know he or she is infected. But there are medical tests that can be given to determine if a person has one of these infections. Females can and should be tested for chlamydia from the first time they have sexual intercourse and every year up to the age of twenty-five. Syphilis is an extremely dangerous STD, and if not treated can result in death. If a test shows that a person has chlamydia, gonorrhoea, or syphilis, that person and their partner should start medical treatment by a doctor or nurse as soon as possible.

Hepatitis is caused by a virus that infects a person's liver. There are many different kinds of hepatitis. Medical tests can determine if a person has hepatitis.

Hepatitis B is an STD that is very contagious. It can be passed on during sexual intercourse and by using unclean needles and syringes. People who take drugs by using or sharing unclean needles and syringes run a big risk of getting this STD. If you have your ears pierced or get a tattoo, you must make sure that a brand-new, germ-free needle is used. There is no cure for hepatitis B, but there is a vaccine that can keep a person from getting the virus. A pregnant woman can pass the virus on to her new baby during birth, so high risk babies (born to mothers with hepatitis B) are given the vaccine.

Hepatitis C can also be spread by sexual contact and passed on by the use of unclean needles and syringes. There is not yet a vaccine for hepatitis C. However, there are treatments a person can take, including pills, which can make it possible for someone who has hepatitis C to be cured.

HPV, an STD caused by a virus called human papilloma-virus, is very contagious and can cause cervical cancer and genital warts. A vaccination – a series of three injections – is given to girls aged twelve to thirteen for free and to people at high risk of contracting the disease. This vaccine prevents females and males from getting or passing on HPV and prevents females from getting cervical cancer. The vaccine works best before a person has any kind of sexual contact.

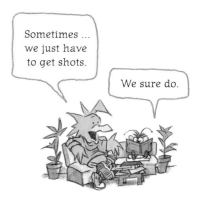

Sometimes ... we just have to get shots.

We sure do.

In some cases HPV goes away on its own. Some females and males can feel genital warts – bumps or growths – on or around their genitals or anus. They may also feel itching. Most do not feel either and do not know they have genital warts. That's why it's important to have regular check-ups. A smear test can determine if a female has HPV on her cervix. A medicine can be applied on the cervix to remove the warts or they can be removed by a doctor.

Herpes simplex virus causes an infection that can be, but is not always, sexually trans-mitted. This virus is passed on from one person to another by skin-to-skin contact and is extremely contagious. Herpes simplex virus can also be spread by saliva.

Herpes 1 causes blister-like sores to form on or near a person's lips, mouth, nose and eyes. Herpes 2, or genital herpes, causes blister-like sores to form on or near a person's genitals and anus. Often people do not know that they have herpes. There are medical tests that can determine if a person has herpes. No cure has been found for the herpes simplex virus, but both types can be treated by a doctor with medicine that can make the sores go away and make the infected area feel better. However, the sores can come back. A pregnant woman can pass the virus to her baby during birth.

It is mostly adults and teenagers who get STDs. If a person has sexual contact, using a new condom correctly and every time can help protect him or her from getting or passing on some of these infections. This is one way of practising safer sex. Unprotected sex is extremely risky.

Condoms are the only contraception that can help to protect one from getting an STD or passing on an STD to another person. Abstinence is the surest way to protect oneself from getting infected by a sexually transmitted disease.

Not all infections are caused by sexual contact.

But if a person feels discomfort or pain on or near any of the sexual parts of his or her body, it is important to tell his or her parent, or the school nurse, or another trusted adult, so that a medical check-up can be arranged. If a person has a sexually transmitted disease, getting prompt medical care may make that person feel better. It may also save his or her life, as well as stop the spread of the infection to another person.

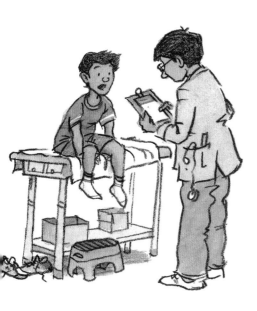

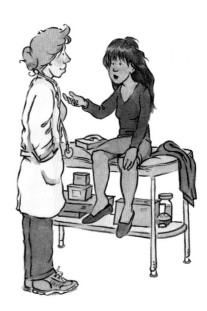

28
Scientists Working Day and Night
HIV and AIDS

HIV infection is a sexually transmitted disease and is the most dangerous of all STDs. HIV is the germ – the virus – that causes AIDS. If a person is infected with another STD, that person has a high risk of becoming infected with HIV as well.

The letters *HIV* stand for *human immunodeficiency virus –* the scientific term for the AIDS virus, HIV. *Virus* means *a type of germ – too small to see without a microscope – that can cause a person to become ill.* The letters *AIDS* stand for *acquired immunodeficiency syndrome –* the scientific term for AIDS. *Acquired* means *something you can get. Immunodeficiency* means *not able to protect against or fight infections and cancer. Syndrome* means *a group of symptoms or conditions that may accompany an illness or a disease.*

What HIV and AIDS mean is that when people who are infected with HIV develop AIDS and become sick, their bodies are no longer able to protect against or fight infections and cancer. Scientists and doctors know that most people who are infected with HIV and do not receive treatment will eventually develop the symptoms or conditions of AIDS. These include coughing, fevers, weight loss, swollen glands, diarrhoea, and being unable to think or see clearly. A person who has HIV infection may not get sick for a long time, as long as ten years or more. However, most people who develop AIDS and do not receive anti-HIV drugs eventually die from one or more of its symptoms or conditions.

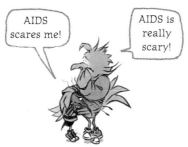

At this time, there is no cure for AIDS. But there are some medicines that can slow down the virus and keep it from spreading in the body for many years. These drugs are helping some HIV-infected people to feel healthier and live long lives.

Any person can get HIV infection – young or old, male or female, rich or poor, straight, gay, lesbian, bisexual, or transgender, famous or not famous, weak or strong. Any person of any race or any religion can get infected with HIV and can develop AIDS. HIV infection has nothing to do with who you are; it can have a lot to do with what you do.

A blood test that doctors and nurses perform shows whether a person has been infected with HIV. If a person has the virus, he or she could remain healthy and lead a good and productive life for many years. Without the blood test, it is not easy to know if the virus is in a person's body. The term *HIV positive* means that a person has HIV infection in his or her body. But scientists and doctors have learned a lot about HIV and have discovered ways a person *cannot* get HIV infection – and ways a person *can* get HIV infection.

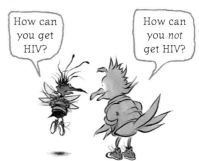

Ways you *cannot* get HIV infection

• You cannot get HIV by playing tag, wrestling, hugging, shaking hands with, dancing with or giving a friendly kiss hello to a person who has HIV.

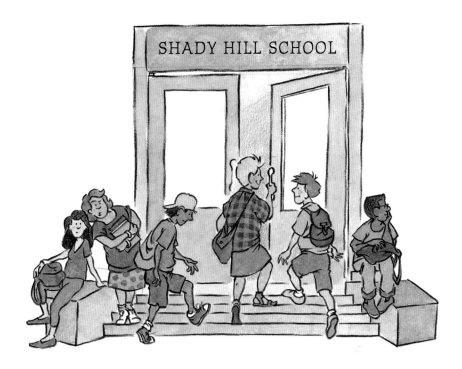

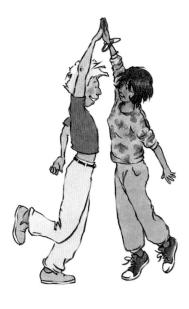

• You cannot get HIV from food, a plate, a doorknob, a comb, a brush, or a toilet seat that a person with HIV has touched.

• You cannot catch HIV the way you catch a cold, because the germ or virus does not travel through the air. That means you cannot get HIV from a cough or a sneeze.

• You cannot get HIV from donating blood.

• You cannot get HIV from a mosquito or flea bite.

• You cannot get HIV just by being in the same room with someone who has HIV. That means you cannot get HIV just by going to school with someone who has HIV.

• You cannot get HIV by swimming in the same pool with someone who has HIV.

• You cannot get HIV from visiting someone who has HIV at home or in the hospital.

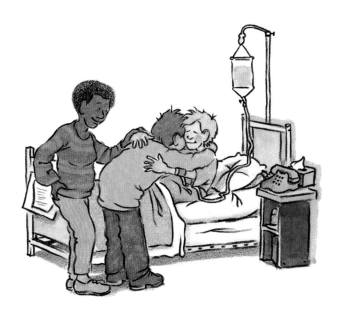

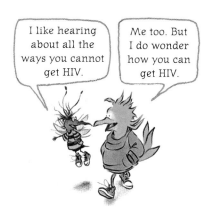

I like hearing about all the ways you cannot get HIV.

Me too. But I do wonder how you can get HIV.

Ways you *can* get HIV infection

- You can get HIV from a person who has the virus either from semen from the male's penis or fluids from the female's vagina. These body fluids carry HIV. That means you can get HIV from having sexual intercourse with a person who is infected with the virus even if that person appears to be healthy.

- It also means that if a person has vaginal sex, oral sex or anal sex with someone who has HIV, and does not protect himself or herself correctly and every time, there is a real risk of getting infected with HIV.

  If a person chooses to have sex, using a new condom every time a person has sex can help protect him or her from getting HIV. Unprotected sex is extremely risky.

- You can get HIV from the blood of a person who has the virus. That means you can get the virus if the blood from a person infected with HIV enters your bloodstream – or if blood that has HIV in it is injected into your body. However, all blood donated for children, babies, and adults who need blood in a hospital or at home is tested to make sure it does not have HIV in it before it is given to them.

- You can get HIV if you take drugs by using a needle and syringe that has been used by a person who has HIV. People who take drugs by using unclean needles and syringes or sharing needles run a big risk of getting HIV.

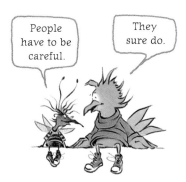

People have to be careful.

They sure do.

But every time you have a jab from your doctor or nurse to keep you healthy, a brand-new, disposable, clean, germ-free, sterile needle and syringe are used and then thrown away in a safe place. You cannot get HIV from brand-new, germ-free needles and syringes. If you have your ears pierced or get a tattoo, you must make sure that the needle used is brand-new, germ-free, and disposable.

- A female who has HIV can pass the virus to her fetus while it is in her uterus, or to her baby during birth. That is why some babies are born with HIV. But a pregnant female can take medicine that can keep her baby from being born with HIV.

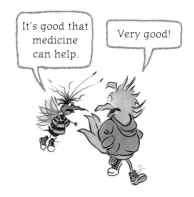

It's good that medicine can help.

Very good!

- Some mothers who have HIV can pass the virus on to their babies through their breast milk. Instead a baby can drink a special drink from a bottle, called formula, which has some milk, vitamins, salt, and sugar in it.

  Luckily, scientists and doctors have discovered ways in which people can protect themselves from getting HIV and lessen their chances of developing AIDS. One way is to abstain from having sexual intercourse with another person. This is called abstinence and is the only fully safe way people can protect themselves from getting HIV through sexual contact.

If a person chooses to have sexual intercourse, using a male condom can lessen his or her chance of getting HIV infection. You may have heard the term "safer sex". Using a new condom correctly and every time is one way people are practising safer sex. Not sharing needles is another way to avoid the chance of getting HIV infection.

Scientists all over the world are working day and night in laboratories to try to make a vaccine that will prevent a

person from being infected with HIV if he or she comes into contact with the virus. Just as there are vaccines to protect people from being infected with measles, mumps or polio, an HIV vaccine could prevent a person from being infected with HIV and developing AIDS.

Scientists are also working on making pills, injections or other treatments that they hope will help people who already have the AIDS virus to lead longer and healthier lives. They hope that such treatments will either keep the virus quiet so that it will not be able to harm a person or will eliminate the

virus from a person's body entirely. Sometimes, these treatments for HIV can make the infected person feel ill. That's why scientists are also working to develop medicines and treatments for HIV that can help make an infected person feel less tired or less uncomfortable.

But even without a vaccine or treatment, people can help protect themselves from getting HIV infection by knowing how the virus is passed from one person to another.

Many people who are HIV positive or who have developed AIDS are able to go to work or school and carry on with most

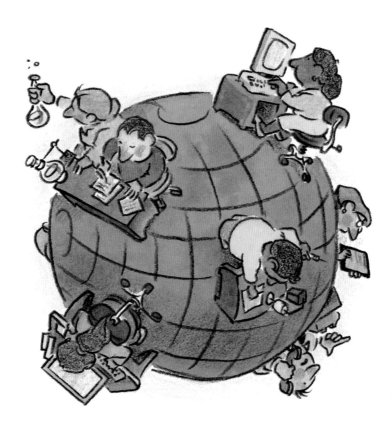

parts of their lives for a number of years, until the virus makes them too ill.

And yet people, both children and adults, who are HIV positive or who have developed AIDS have been discriminated against. Some children, along with their families, have been forced to move – only because they are HIV positive or have developed AIDS.

Having HIV infection as well as developing AIDS is sad and painful in many ways. So, if you know someone who is HIV positive or has developed AIDS, treat that person kindly. Shake hands, say hello, give a hug, talk with that person, laugh and even cry with that person, and work and play with that person – all these things are safe to do – and treat that person as you would treat any good friend.

29
Staying Healthy
Responsible Choices

A large part of growing up is learning to take care of yourself in a healthy way.

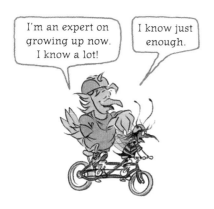

I'm an expert on growing up now. I know a lot!

I know just enough.

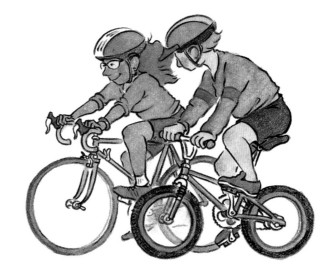

Eating healthy foods, exercising almost daily, keeping your body clean, wearing clean clothes, staying away from drugs and alcohol, and having regular medical check-ups – all of these things can help you be healthy and stay healthy as you go through puberty.

But there's more to staying healthy than just taking good care of your body. It also means taking responsibility for your own actions – for yourself and for what you do. It means making healthy choices for yourself, including choices about your body and about sex. And it means having respect for yourself and your own decisions.

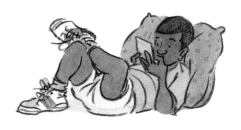

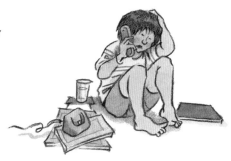

Staying healthy also involves having healthy relationships with other people. That means not only taking good care of yourself, but taking good care of your friends – both boys and girls. Having a good friend or friends as you grow up can help you learn how to have healthy relationships with other people that involve sharing, caring and respect for others as well as for yourself.

As you go through life, friendship is a big part of every healthy relationship, whether two people like, love, or like and love each other, whether they choose to be friends, to date, to be partners or to marry.

Yet puberty is a time when friends, even good friends, often try to persuade or pressure each other to try out new things. Some of these things, which may involve sex, alcohol or drugs, may be things you do not want to do, or are not ready to do, or are afraid to do, or feel are not safe to do. That's when it's important to make the decision that is best

for you – one that is safe and healthy for you.

Everyone makes mistakes and has bad judgement once in a while, and you probably will too. But most of the time, you can and will make responsible choices – ones that are good for you, right for you, and healthy for you and your friends.

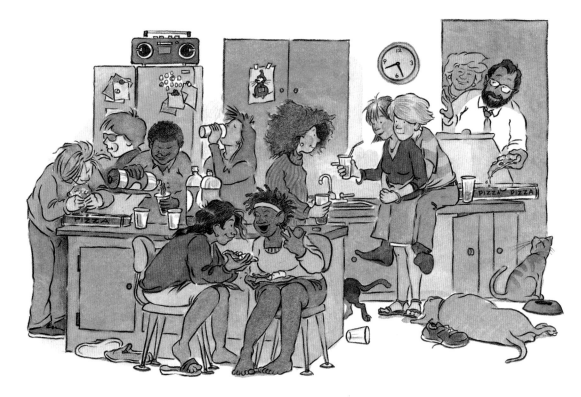

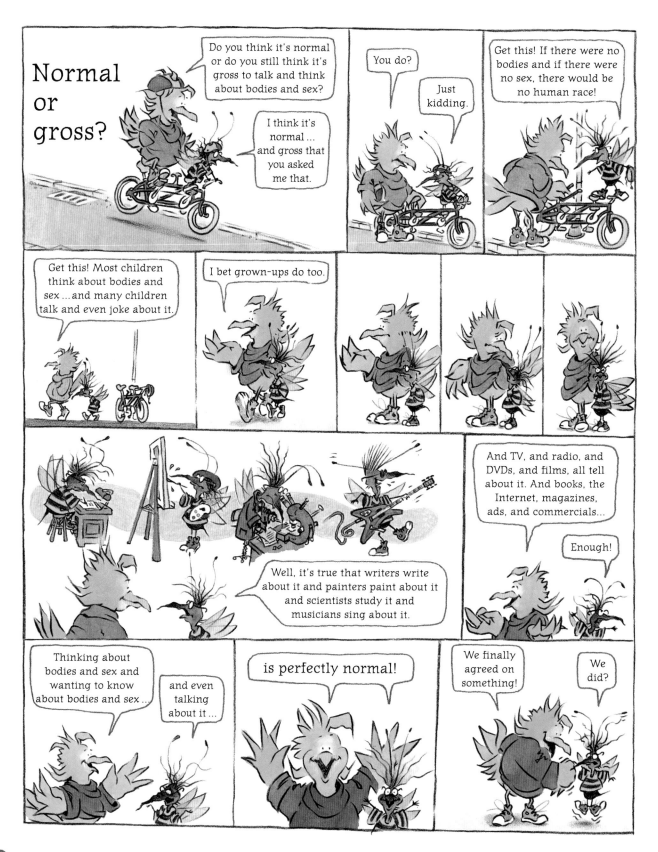

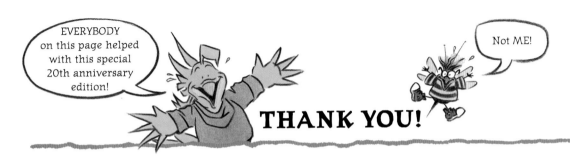

EVERYBODY on this page helped with this special 20th anniversary edition!

Not ME!

THANK YOU!

Without all of you, we could not have created this newest edition of *Let's Talk About Sex*. Your expertise helped us ensure that this book contains the latest and most accurate information possible – information that can help today's children and teens stay healthy. Thank you for teaching us so well.

R. H. H. and M. E.

Bebe J. Anderson, JD, *director, U.S. Legal Program, Center for Reproductive Rights, New York, NY*

Wendy Apfel, *educational technology coordinator, Bank Street School for Children, New York, NY*

Joan E. Bertin, JD, *executive director, National Coalition Against Censorship, New York, NY*

Deborah Chamberlain, MA, LMHC, *mental health specialist, Cambridge, MA*

Angela Diaz, MD, MPH, *professor, Department of Pediatrics and Department of Preventative Medicine, Icahn School of Medicine at Mount Sinai, director, Mount Sinai Adolescent Health Center, New York, NY*

Benjamin H. Harris, PhD, *clinical psychologist, Doctoral Program in Clinical Psychology, City College @ CUNY, New York, NY*

David B. Harris, PhD, *child advocate, Children's Research and Education Institute, New York, NY*

Emily B. Harris, MD, *pediatrician, New York, NY*

Hilary G. Harris, *parent, New York, NY*

William W. Harris, PhD, *child advocate, Children's Research and Education Institute, New York, NY*

Alexandra M. Harrison, MD, *child psychiatrist, child and adult psychoanalyst, Boston Psychoanalytic Society and Institute; Cambridge Health Alliance, Cambridge, MA*

Robyn Heilbrun, JD, *consultant, Sausalito, CA*

Jennifer Johnsen, MPH, *director of health information, Planned Parenthood Federation of America, New York, NY*

Leslie M. Kantor, MPH, *vice president of education, Planned Parenthood Federation of America; assistant professor, Mailman School of Public Health, Columbia University, New York, NY*

Perri Klass, MD, *professor of journalism and pediatrics, New York University, New York, NY*

Susan Kuklin, *children's book author and photographer, New York, NY*

Elizabeth A. Levy, *children's book author, New York, NY*

Jay A. Levy, MD, *professor, Department of Medicine, research associate, Cancer Research Institute, University of California School of Medicine, San Francisco, CA*

Benjamin Lowengard, *technical consultant, Belmont, MA*

Nancy Meyer, *parent, New York, NY*

Eli H. Newberger, MD, *pediatrician; founder and medical director, 1970–2000, Child Protection Program; Adjunct in Pediatrics, Boston Children's Hospital; Assistant Professor of Pediatrics, Harvard Medical School, Boston, MA*

Heather Z. Sankey, MD, *vice chair for education, Department of Obstetrics and Gynecology, Baystate Medical Center, Springfield, MA*

Annabel Sheinberg, MM, *education director, Planned Parenthood Association of Utah, Salt Lake City, UT*

Norman Spack, MD, *co-director, Gender Management Service, Endocrine Division, Boston Children's Hospital, Boston, MA*

Marc N. Weiss, *Web Lab, New York, NY*

A giant thank-you to our editor, **Hilary Van Dusen,** *our designer,* **Nathan Pyritz,** *and our art director,* **Chris Paul,** *for your commitment to keeping this book current for today's children and teens, no matter how much time and work it took to do so.*

THANK YOU!

Ever since we first created this book, we could not have written, illustrated, and updated it whenever we needed to without the help of the following old and new friends and colleagues. Some read the whole manuscript; others read only a chapter. Some read the manuscript once; others read it numerous times. Many helped with the drawings. Everyone had something to say about this book and answered any question we had, often more than once. The people listed here all have one thing in common. They care deeply about the health and well-being of children and have enormous respect for children.

R. H. H. and M. E.

Deb Allen, *elementary school science coordinator and teacher, The Devotion School, Brookline, MA*

Tina Alu, *sexuality education coordinator, Cambridge Family Planning, Cambridge, MA*

Joanne Amico, *health educator, Pierce School, Brookline, MA*

Bonnie S. Anderson, PhD, *professor of history, Brooklyn College, Brooklyn, NY*

Fran Basch, *professional trainer, Planned Parenthood League of MA, Cambridge, MA*

Merton Bernfield, MD, *Clement A. Smith Professor of Pediatrics, director, Joint Program in Neonatology, Children's Hospital, Boston, MA*

Sarah Birss, MD, *child psychiatrist, developmental pediatrician, Cambridge, MA*

Larry Boggess, *school administrator, writer, Richmond, IN*

Alice Miller Bregman, *senior editor, New York, NY*

Rosa Casamassima, *consultant, Medford, MA*

Deborah Chamberlain, MA, LMHC, *mental health specialist, Cambridge, MA*

David S. Chapin, MD, *director of gynecology, Beth Israel Hospital, Boston, MA*

Chuck and Paula Collins, *parents, San Francisco, CA*

Edward J. Collins, MD, *assistant clinical professor, University of California at San Francisco, CA*

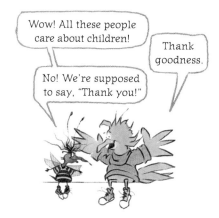

Wow! All these people care about children!

No! We're supposed to say, "Thank you!"

Thank goodness.

Julia Collins, *student, San Francisco, CA*

Sara Collins, *student, San Francisco, CA*

Sally Crissman, *science educator, Shady Hill School, Cambridge, MA*

Mollianne Cunniff, *health educator, Brookline Public Schools, Brookline, MA*

Kirsten Dahl, PhD, *associate professor, Yale University Child Study Center, New Haven, CT*

Angela Diaz, MD, MPH, *professor Department of Pediatrics and Department of Preventative Medicine, Icahn School of Medicine at Mount Sinai, director, Mount Sinai Adolescent Health Center, New York, NY*

Mary Dominguez, *science teacher, Shady Hill School, Cambridge, MA*

Catherine Donagher, *parent, Brookline, MA*

Sheila Donelan, *teacher, M. E. Fitzgerald School, Cambridge, MA*

Sandra Downes, *teacher, Amos E. Lawrence School, Brookline, MA*

Nancy Drooker, *sexuality education consultant, San Francisco, CA*

Dan Frank, PhD, *principal, Francis W. Parker School, Chicago, IL*

Nicki Nichols Gamble, *consultant, Cambridge, MA*

Frieda Garcia, *president, United South End Settlements, Boston, MA*

Judith Gardner, PhD, *psychologist, Brandeis University, Waltham, MA*

Trudy Goodman, MEd, *child and family therapist, Cambridge, MA*

Benjamin H. Harris, PhD, *clinical psychologist, Doctoral Program in Clinical Psychology, City College @ CUNY, New York, NY*

David B. Harris, PhD, *child advocate, Children's Research and Education Institute, New York, NY*

William W. Harris, PhD, *child advocate, Children's Research and Education Institute, New York, NY*

Emily B. Harris, MD, *pediatrician, New York, NY*

William Haseltine, PhD, *chief, Division of Human Retrovirology, Harvard Medical School, Dana Farber Cancer Institute, Boston, MA*

Gerald Hass, MD, *pediatrician, Cambridge, MA; physician in chief, South End Community Health Center, Boston, MA*

M. Peter Heilbrun, MD, *chairman, Department of Neurosurgery, University of Utah, Salt Lake City, UT*

Robyn O. Heilbrun, *parent, Salt Lake City, UT*

Doris B. Held, MEd, *psychotherapist, Harvard Medical School; member of the Governor's Commission on Gay and Lesbian Youth for the Commonwealth of MA, Cambridge, MA*

Michael Iskowitz, *chief counsel for poverty, AIDS, and family policy, U.S. Senate Committee on Labor and Human Resources, Washington, D.C.*

Chris Jagmin, *designer, Watertown, MA*

Susan Kaitz, *director of health education, Newton Public Schools, Newton, MA*

Leslie M. Kantor, MPH, *vice president of education, Planned Parenthood Federation of America; assistant professor, Mailman School of Public Health, Columbia University, New York, NY*

Jill Kantrowitz, *director of education, Planned Parenthood of Massachusetts, Boston, MA*

Larry Kessler, *executive director, AIDS Action Committee of MA, Boston, MA; commissioner, U.S. National Commission on AIDS, Washington, D.C.*

Robert A. King, MD, *assistant professor of child psychiatry, Yale University Child Study Center, New Haven, CT*

Peri Klass, MD, *professor of journalism and pediatrics, New York University, New York, NY*

Antoinette E. M. Leoney, Esq., *parent, Salem, MA*

Elizabeth A. Levy, *children's book author, New York, NY*

Jay Levy, MD, *professor, Department of Medicine, research associate, Cancer Research Institute, University of California School of Medicine at San Francisco, CA*

Leroy Lewis, *teacher, Martin Luther King School, Cambridge, MA*

Carol Lynch, *director of counseling, Planned Parenthood Clinic, Brookline, MA*

Lyn Marshall, *teacher, The Atrium School, Watertown, MA*

Michael McGee, *vice president for education, Planned Parenthood Federation of America, New York, NY*

Kristin Mercer, *student, Arlington, MA*

Ted Mermin, *teacher, The Atrium School, Watertown, MA*

Ronald James Moglia, EdD, *director, Graduate Program in Human Sexuality, New York University, New York, NY*

Rory Jay Morton, *teacher, Shady Hill School, Cambridge, MA*

Eli Newberger, MD, *director, Family Development Program, Children's Hospital, Boston, MA*

Brenda O'Conner, *teacher, M. E. Fitzgerald School, Cambridge, MA*

Dian Olson, *educator and trainer, Planned Parenthood League of MA, Cambridge, MA*

June E. Osborn, MD, *dean, School of Public Health, University of Michigan; chairman, U.S. National Commission on AIDS, Washington, D.C.*

Jimmy Parziale, *teacher, Michael Driscoll School, Brookline, MA*

Kyle Pruett, MD, *clinical professor of psychiatry, Yale University Child Study Center, New Haven, CT*

Jeffrey Pudney, PhD, *research associate, Harvard Medical School, Boston, MA*

Frank W. Putnam, MD, *professor of pediatrics and psychiatry, Cincinnati Children's Hospital Medical Center, Cincinnati, OH*

Jennifer Quest-Stern, *student, Cambridge, MA*

Louise Rice, RN, *associate director of education, AIDS Action Committee of Massachusetts, Boston, MA*

Monica Rodriguez, *director of information and education, Sexuality Information and Education Council of the United States, New York, NY*

Charles D. Roos, *consultant, New York, NY*

Sukey Rosenbaum, *parent, New York, NY*

Deborah M. Rothman, *sexuality educator, author, Baltimore, MD*

Heather Z. Sankey, MD, *vice chair for education, Department of Obstetrics and Gynecology, Baystate Medical Center, Springfield, MA*

Kate Seeger, *teacher, Shady Hill School, Cambridge, MA*

Rachel Skvirsky, PhD, *associate professor of biology, University of Massachusetts, Boston, MA*

Priscilla J. Smith, JD, *director, Domestic Legal Program, Center for Reproductive Rights, New York, NY*

Paula Stahl, EdD, *executive director, Children's Charter Trauma Clinic, Waltham, MA*

Michael G. Thompson, PhD, *clinical psychologist, author, Cambridge, MA*

Laurence H. Tribe, *Tyler Professor of Constitutional Law, Harvard Law School, Cambridge, MA*

Maeve Visser Knoth, *librarian, San Mateo County Library, Atherton, CA*

Polly Wagner, *teacher, The Atrium School, Watertown, MA*

Lilla Waltch, *author, Cambridge, MA*

Susan Webber, *consultant, Arlington, MA*

Rosalind M. Weir, *parent, Cambridge, MA*

Ilyon Woo, *student, Cambridge, MA*

Donna Yee, PhD, *consultant, Visions Inc., Cambridge, MA*

Barry Zuckerman, MD, *professor of pediatrics, Boston University School of Medicine, Boston, MA*

Pamela Zuckerman, MD, *pediatrician, Boston, MA*

A special thank-you to our editor, **Amy Ehrlich,** *for her wholehearted commitment to this book and her courage for taking it on; to our art director,* **Virginia Evans,** *for listening to us and seeing our vision; to our associate editor,* **Jane Snyder,** *for keeping track of every word and everyone; to their colleagues at* **Candlewick Press** *for their enthusiastic support; to our agent,* **Elaine Markson,** *for her friendship and belief in this book; and to our designer,* **Lance Hidy,** *for his brilliant eye and pitch-perfect design; and special thanks to* **Mary Lee Donovan, Andrea Tompa, Hilary Van Dusen,** *and* **Caroline Lawrence.**

INDEX

A

abortion 71–3
Abortion Act (1967) 72
abstinence 50, 52, 53, 65–6, 70, 85
    and HIV prevention 88–9
Adam's apple 37
adolescence 25
    see also puberty
adoption 45, 63–4
    birth parents 48, 64
AIDS 7, 75, 86, 88–90
amniotic fluid/sac 56, 58, 60
anal sex 53, 65, 69
ancient Greece 8–9
anus 17, 20
artificial insemination 62, 63
athletic box 39

B

babies
    birth 18, 58–61
    birth weight 46
    and families 45–7
    first cry 60
    and HIV 88
    multiple births 49
    ovaries of baby girls 18
    and sex chromosomes 49
    and teenage parents 46–7
    see also pregnancy
birth control (contraception) 52,
    66–70
birth parents 48, 64
bisexual people 9, 10–11
blood
    and HIV 88
    menstrual 29
bodies 12–15
    growth spurts 36, 37
    sex organs 3–4
        females 3, 4, 16–18
        males 3, 4, 19–21
    and sexual abuse 80, 81–2
    and sexual reproduction 3–4, 6, 18,
    27
    size of body parts 40
    talking about 22–3
    see also puberty
boys *see* males

bras 39
breast milk 88
breasts 36
    bras 39
    size of 40
breech births 58, 60

C

Caesarean births (c-sections) 58–60
cervical cancer 84
cervical cap 67, 69
cervix 18, 69
chlamydia 67, 83–4
chromosomes 48, 49
circumcision 19, 60–1
clitoris 16, 44
"coming" *see* orgasm
conception (fertilized eggs) 27, 32, 48,
    54–5
condoms 66–7, 69, 85
    and safer sex 52, 53, 67, 88, 89
contraception 52, 66–70
crushes 5, 10
cyber bullying 79

D

diaphragm 67, 69
dirty jokes 22, 23
DNA 48
doctors
    and abortion 71, 72, 73
    and alternative methods of
    conception 62–3
    and the birth of a baby 58, 60
    and contraception 66, 67, 70
    physical examinations by 81
    and puberty 39
        menstruation 29
    and sexually transmitted diseases
    84
        HIV/AIDS 86, 88–9
dreams 44
drugs 57
    anti HIV 86
    and sexually transmitted diseases
    84

E

egg cells (ova) 18
    and chromosomes 48
    and contraception 68, 69–70
    fertilization 27, 32, 48
        conception 27, 54–5
        failure of 62
        and genes 48
        and twins 49
    frozen 63
    and menstruation 27–8, 29
    and puberty 27
    and surrogate pregnancies 63
ejaculation 21, 32, 33, 34–5, 37
    and conception 54, 55
    and contraception 70
    and sexual intercourse 51, 54, 55
embryos 54, 56
emergency contraception 69
epididymis 21, 32, 33, 34
erections 19, 32–4

F

faces
    facial hair in boys 37, 38
    oiliness and spots 38–9
    puberty changes in 36, 37
faeces (solid waste) 17, 20
Fallopian tubes 18, 27, 28
    and conception 54, 55
    and sterilization 70
families
    and babies 45–7, 58
    and body changes in puberty 40–1
    family members 45
    genes and chromosomes 48–9
    and sexual abuse 80–1
feelings
    changes in puberty 40–1
    sexual desire 4–5
    sexual feelings 43
    and sexual intercourse 6, 7
female condoms 67
females 2–3
    bodies 14, 15
        sex organs 3, 4, 16–18
    bras 39
    contraception 67–70
    masturbation 44

puberty 18, 24, 25, 26, 27–31
    changes in 36, 37, 38, 39
    and sex chromosomes 49
    and sexually transmitted diseases
    84
    see also menstruation
fetuses 18, 54, 55, 56–7
forceps births 58, 60
fraternal twins 49
friendships
    healthy 91
    and HIV 90
    and puberty 41–2

G

gay (homosexual) people 8–11, 45
gender 3, 49
genes 48, 49
genital herpes 85
genital warts 84
girls *see* females
gonorrhoea 52, 53, 83–4

H

hair in puberty
    growth 36, 37, 38
    oily hair 36, 37, 38, 39
hard ons (erections) 19, 32–4
having sex *see* sexual intercourse
health 39, 90–1
    and pregnancy 57
    sexual health and the Internet 75
hepatitis B 66, 67, 84
hepatitis C 84
herpes 84–5
heterosexual (straight) 8
hips 36
HIV 86–90
    prevention 66, 67
    and sexual intercourse 7, 52, 53, 88
    treatments 89
    ways you can get 88
    ways you cannot get 87
    website information on 75
homosexual (gay) people 8–11, 45
hormones 25–6, 27, 32
    and mood swings 42
HPV 52, 53, 84
Human Fertilization and Embryology
    Act (1990) 72
hymen 17

I

identical twins 49
implants, contraceptive 67–8
in vitro fertilization 62, 63
infections *see* sexually transmitted
    diseases (STDs)
injections, contraceptive 68–9
instant messaging 77
Internet safety 74–9
IUDs/IUSs 67, 69

J

jockstraps 39
jokes about bodies and sex 22, 23

L

labia 16
labour (birth) 58
larynx (voice box) 37
lesbians 8–9, 45
LGBT people 10–11

M

making love *see* sexual intercourse
male condoms 52, 53, 66–7, 89
males 2–3
    bodies 14, 15
        sex organs 3, 4, 19–21
    circumcision 19, 60–1
    contraception 66, 69–70
    jockstraps 39
    masturbation 44
    puberty 20, 24, 25, 26, 32–5
        changes in 37
        and ejaculation 21
    and sex chromosomes 49
    sex organs 3, 4, 19–21
    vasectomies 70
    see also sperm
masturbation 43–4
menopause 29
menstruation (having a period) 18,
    27–31, 36
    and egg cells 27–8, 29
    first periods 29, 30–1
    irregular periods 29
    the menstrual cycle 29
    and pregnancy 29, 36, 46, 52
    sanitary towels and tampons
    29–30, 31
    talking about 30–1

midwives 59, 60
miscarriages 73
mobile phones 74, 79
mood swings in puberty 42
morning-after pills 69

N

navel (tummy button) 60
nipples 36, 37
"No", right to say 7, 51, 81, 82
nocturnal emissions (wet dreams) 35
nurses 29, 70

O

oestrogen 27
oral sex 53, 65
orgasms 34, 44, 51, 52
ovaries 4, 18
    and puberty 26, 27, 36
ovulation 27

P

pads, menstrual 29–30
parents
    adoption 63–4
    and genes 48
    newborn babies 60, 61
    teenage parents 46–7
patches, contraceptive 68, 69
penis 4, 19, 20, 37
    circumcision 19, 60–1
    erections 19, 32–4
    foreskin 19, 61
    and hair growth 37, 38
    masturbation 44
    and sexual intercourse 7, 8, 18, 51
    size of 40
    and the urethra 21
    see also ejaculation
periods (menstruation) 18
pills
    abortion 71
    contraceptive 67, 68
    morning-after 69
placenta 56–7, 58, 60
pornography 76
postponement of sex 50, 65–6, 70
pregnancy 54–7
    giving birth 18, 58–61
    and HIV 88
    and menstruation 29, 36, 46, 52

and sexual intercourse 7, 29, 35, 37, 51, 52, 53
and sexually transmitted diseases 84, 85
surrogate 63
premature births (prem babies) 61
progesterone 27
prostate gland 32, 34
puberty 24–44
  age of starting 18, 20, 24, 25, 40–1
  celebration of 26
  changes 36–42
    and care of the body 38–9
    in feelings 40–1
  and hormones 25–6, 27, 32
  staying healthy 39, 90–1
  website information on 75
  see also females; males
pubic hair 36, 37, 38
pubic lice 83

R

rape 69, 71
religions 19, 38, 43, 61, 70
rhythm method of birth control 69–70
ring, contraceptive 68–9
rubbers (condoms) 52, 53, 66–7

S

safer sex 52–3, 85, 89
safety on the Internet 74–9
sanitary towels 29–30, 31
Sappho 8–9
scabies 83
scrotum 19, 20, 32, 37
semen 21, 32
  ejaculation 21, 32, 33, 34–5, 37
    and sexual intercourse 51, 52
seminal vesicles 32, 33, 34
sex organs see bodies
sexting 78
sexual abuse 80–2
sexual feelings
  desire 4–5
  and masturbation 43–4
  and sexual intercourse 50–1
sexual health clinics 70
sexual intercourse 6–7, 50–3
  anal 53, 65, 69
  condom use 66–7
  and contraception 66
  and ejaculation 35

and erections 34
and HIV 7, 52, 53, 88
oral 53, 65
postponement of 50, 65–6, 70
and pregnancy 7, 29, 35, 37, 51, 52, 53
right to say "No" 51
and sexually transmitted diseases 83, 84
  HIV 88, 89
see also vaginal intercourse
sexuality 7
sexually transmitted diseases (STDs) 7, 65, 66, 75, 83–90
shaving 38
slang words 22
social network sites 75, 77
solid waste (faeces) 17, 20
Sparta 9
sperm 20, 21, 32
  artificial insemination 62, 63
  and chromosomes 48
  and fertilized eggs 27, 48, 54
  puberty and sperm production 26, 32
  and surrogate pregnancies 63
  see also ejaculation
spermicides 69
spots (zits) 38–9
stepparents 45
sterilization 70
STIs see sexually transmitted diseases (STDs)
straight (heterosexual) 8, 9
surrogate pregnancies 63
sweating in puberty 36, 37, 38
syphilis 83–4

T

talking
  about bodies and sex 22–3
  and sexual abuse 81
tampons 29–30, 31
teasing 41, 42
testicles 4, 19, 20, 21
  and puberty 26, 32, 37
testosterone 32, 33
texting 74, 77, 78–9
touching 50, 51
transgender people 10–11
tummy button (naval) 60
twins 49

U

umbilical cord 57, 59, 60
urethra
  female body 16, 17
  male body 21, 32
urine (liquid waste) 17, 19, 21, 35
uterus (womb) 17, 18
  and conception 27, 54, 55
  and menstruation 27, 28
  pregnancy 54, 56
    and birth 58, 59, 60

V

vagina 4, 17, 18
  and the birth of a baby 18, 58, 59
  and contraception 67, 69
  and menstruation 18, 27
  vaginal fluid 36
vaginal intercourse 7, 8, 18, 51, 51–2, 65
  and contraception 66, 69–70
vas deferens 21, 32, 33, 34, 70
vasectomies 70
vulva 16

W

washing 38
wet dreams 35
withdrawal method of birth control 69, 70

X, Y

X and Y chromosomes 49

Z

zits (spots) 38–9
zygotes 54, 56

To my husband,
to my children, to Val.
Thanks, guys!
R.H.H.

To my parents
M.E.

First published in Great Britain 1994 by Walker Books Ltd
87 Vauxhall Walk, London SE11 5HJ

This edition published 2014

2 4 6 8 10 9 7 5 3 1

Text © 1994, 2004, 2009, 2014 by BEE Productions, Inc.
Illustrations © 1994, 2004, 2009, 2014 by BIRD Productions, Inc.

The right of Robie Harris and Michael Emberley to be identified as author and illustrator of this work
has been asserted by them in accordance with the Copyright, Designs and Patents Act 1988

This book was typeset in Stempel Schneidler and Journal.

Printed in China

British Library Cataloguing in Publication Data:
a catalogue record for this book is available from the British Library

ISBN 978-1-4063-5604-5

www.walker.co.uk

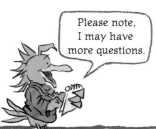

NOTES

NOTES

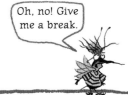

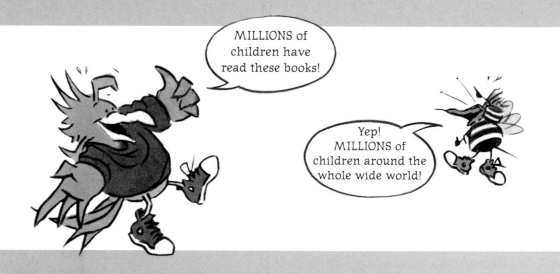
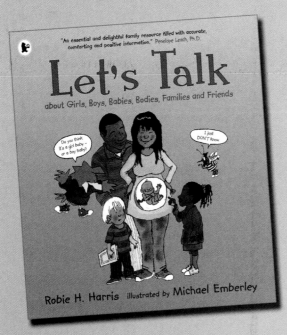

Let's Talk About Where Babies Come From

provides accurate, unbiased answers to nearly every conceivable question about reproduction, birth, and babies, while giving children a healthy understanding of their bodies.

"It is non-judgemental but responsible, giving children enough information and social guidance to dispel ignorance and fear, but not too much to leave them exposed or overwhelmed." – *The Times Educational Supplement*

For age **7** *and up*

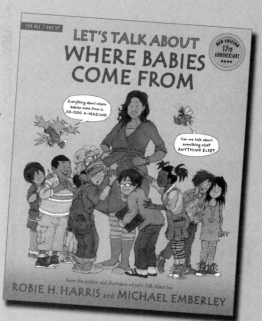

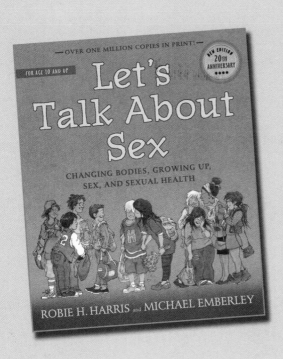

Let's Talk About Sex

offers young people the real information they need to make responsible decisions that can help them stay healthy as they approach and experience puberty and adolescence.

"Brave and comprehensive." – *Guardian*

For age **10** *and up*

Robie H. Harris began her career as a teacher at the Bank Street College of Education's School for Children. Her interest in child development issues and the experience of being a parent made her realize "how difficult but necessary it is to talk with children and teenagers about sex and answer questions about this complicated topic. I wanted my children to stay healthy, so I had to give them accurate information. When I was writing this book, consultations with young people, parents, educators, librarians, doctors, nurses, psychologists, scientists, and members of the clergy confirmed the need to educate our young people about sexual health." Robie H. Harris has received Planned Parenthood Federation of America's highest education award – the Mary Lee Tatum Award. This annual award is given to the person who most exemplifies the qualities of an ideal sexuality educator. She is also the author of *Let's Talk* and *Let's Talk About Where Babies Come From*, both illustrated by Michael Emberley, as well as *Who Has What?*, *Who's In My Family?*, *What's In There?*, and *What's So Yummy?* Robie H. Harris lives in New York City.

Michael Emberley, the son of children's book illustrator Ed Emberley, attended the Rhode Island School of Design. He has been writing and illustrating award-winning books for children for more than thirty years. His titles include *Let's Talk* and *Let's Talk About Where Babies Come From* – both written by Robie H. Harris. About his collaboration with her on *Let's Talk About Sex*, he says, "We felt the same way about the subject from the beginning. Both of us have a strong belief in spreading healthy information rather than hiding it." Michael Emberley lives in Ireland.

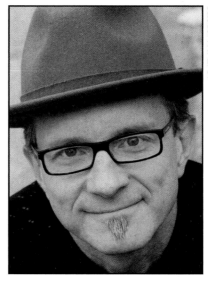